No
GALLBLADDER DIET
Cookbook

Discover the delicious recipes cookbook that offers flavorful solutions for those without a gallbladder, ensuring digestive ease and culinary delight in every meal!

Isabella Abrams

Contents

INTRODUCTION 1

Thriving Without a Gallbladder: Your Guide to Life Post-Surgery.................................1

Nurturing Your Gallbladder Health: Tips for Optimal Digestion...........................1

Strategies for Reducing Gallbladder Attacks and Managing Pain...........................2

Natural Remedies for Promoting Digestive Wellness After Gallbladder Removal 2

Navigating Life After Gallbladder Surgery: A Comprehensive Guide to Health and Well-being 3

Foods to Embrace and Foods to Avoid After Gallbladder Removal 4

Embracing the Benefits of a Thoughtful Diet After Gallbladder Removal 5

Common Questions and Expert Answers for Your Post-Gallbladder Diet Journey 6

The Non-Gallbladder Diet Essentials: Serving Size Guidelines and Meal Planning Principles 7

BREAKFAST...................8

Creamy Oatmeal with Fresh Berries 8

Scrambled Eggs with Spinach and Feta 8

Banana Walnut Pancakes.........................9

Greek Yogurt Parfait 9

Apple Cinnamon Quinoa Porridge 10

Avocado Toast with Poached Eggs 10

Sweet Potato Hash with Turkey Sausage 11

Blueberry Chia Pudding..........................11

Spinach and Mushroom Breakfast Burrito 12

Cottage Cheese and Fruit Bowl 12

Quinoa Breakfast Bowl with Almonds and Honey ...13

Zucchini and Carrot Fritters 13

Veggie Ham and Cheese Omelette 14

Baked Apples with Cinnamon and Almonds........14

Turkey and Veggie Breakfast Casserole 15

Smoked Salmon and Cucumber Breakfast Wrap....15

Spinach and Sun-Dried Tomato Quiche Cups.......16

SALADS........................17

Grilled Chicken and Mixed Greens Salad...........17

Quinoa and Roasted Vegetable Salad 17

Tuna and White Bean Salad 18

Spinach and Strawberry Salad 18

Cucumber and Tomato Salad with Dill Yogurt Dressing 19

Mango and Avocado Salad......................19

Chickpea and Cucumber Salad 20

Kale and Pomegranate Salad....................20

Roasted Beet and Goat Cheese Salad............21

Broccoli and Cranberry Salad 21

Pear and Walnut Salad 22

Asian-Inspired Chicken Salad....................22

Roasted Butternut Squash and Quinoa Salad.......23

Egg Salad with Greens.........................23

Black Bean and Corn Salad......................24

Mediterranean Cucumber and Feta Salad.........24

SNACKS 26

Trail Mix with Nuts and Dried Fruit...............26

Carrot and Cucumber Sticks with Tzatziki Dip 26

Cherry Tomatoes with Fresh Mozzarella...........27

Celery Stuffed with Cream Cheese and Raisins 27

Spinach and Feta Stuffed Mushrooms 27

Yogurt and Cucumber Dip with Pita Wedges 28

Edamame with Sea Salt 28

Roasted Chickpeas 29

Cucumber and Avocado Sushi Rolls 29

Carrot and Hummus Pinwheels 30

Pear and Almond Butter Sandwiches 31

Rice Cake with Avocado and Tomato 31

Cantaloupe and Prosciutto Skewers 32

Tomato and Basil Bruschetta.................. 32

Pineapple and Cottage Cheese Bowls............ 33

FISH AND SEAFOOD RECIPES 34

Baked Lemon Herb Salmon 34

Grilled Shrimp Skewers...................... 34

Baked Cod with Tomato and Basil............... 35

Lemon Garlic Butter Scallops.................. 35

Poached Tilapia with Herbed Yogurt............. 36

Salmon and Asparagus Foil Packets............. 36

Lime Cilantro Shrimp Tacos 37

Lime Herb-Crusted Halibut 37

Baked Teriyaki Salmon 38

Seared Scallops with Mango Salsa 39

Broiled Lemon Pepper Haddock................. 39

Shrimp and Vegetable Stir-Fry 40

Baked Coconut-Crusted Tilapia 41

Salmon and Spinach Stuffed Mushrooms 41

Cilantro Lime Grilled Swordfish 42

Baked Garlic Herb Mussels................... 42

Herb-Crusted Mahi-Mahi..................... 43

Lemon Pepper Baked Snapper.................. 43

Herbed Sea Bass with Cherry Tomatoes.......... 44

POULTRY AND MEAT RECIPES 45

Lemon Herb Grilled Chicken Breast.............. 45

Stuffed Bell Peppers with Lean Ground Beef 45

Herb-Crusted Chicken Thighs.................. 46

Orange Glazed Chicken Drumsticks 46

Cilantro Lime Grilled Turkey Burgers 47

Lemon Garlic Roasted Chicken Thighs 48

Honey Mustard Glazed Turkey Breast 48

Stuffed Zucchini with Ground Chicken 49

Baked Garlic Herb Turkey Meatballs 49

Rosemary and Garlic Roasted Beef Tenderloin 50

Grilled Herb-Marinated Quail 50

Braised Rabbit with Tomato and Herbs........... 51

Grilled Rabbit Skewers with Lemon and Garlic...... 52

Baked Quail with Apricot Glaze 52

Braised Veal with Tomato and Herbs 53

Quail Stuffed with Quinoa and Vegetables 53

Quail and Mushroom Skewers 54

Veal Medallions in Lemon Caper Sauce 54

Braised Beef with Tomatoes and Herbs 55

VEGETARIAN RECIPES 56

Spinach and Quinoa Stuffed Bell Peppers 56

Sweet Potato and Lentil Curry 56

Zucchini Noodles with Pesto 57

Creamy Mushroom Risotto.................... 57

Baked Eggplant Parmesan 58

Cauliflower and Broccoli Bake 59

Grilled Portobello Mushrooms with Balsamic Glaze . 59

Ratatouille............................... 60

Roasted Butternut Squash and Apple Salad........ 61

Cucumber and Dill Greek Yogurt Dip 61

Spinach and Feta Stuffed Tomatoes 62

Roasted Brussels Sprouts with Maple Dijon Glaze .. 62

Eggplant and Chickpea Curry.................. 63

Sweet Potato and Black Bean Tacos............. 64

SOUPS 65

Butternut Squash Soup 65

Lentil and Vegetable Soup 65

Creamy Potato Leek Soup.................... 66

Tomato Basil Soup......................... 67

Mushroom Barley Soup...................... 67

Minestrone Soup 68

Cauliflower and Broccoli Soup 68

Sweet Potato and Ginger Soup. 69

Spinach and Rice Soup 70

Vegan Split Pea Soup 70

Red Lentil and Spinach Soup 71

Zucchini and Basil Soup 71

Pea and Mint Soup. 72

Asparagus and Potato Soup. 72

Cabbage and White Bean Soup 73

Beet and Carrot Soup. 74

SMOOTHIES 75

Banana Berry Bliss. 75

Mango Tango Smoothie 75

Green Detox Smoothie. 76

Pineapple Coconut Delight 76

Avocado and Spinach Smoothie 77

Blueberry Almond Protein Smoothie 77

Peachy Keen Smoothie 78

Cucumber Mint Cooler 78

Carrot Cake Smoothie 79

Cherry Almond Bliss 79

Strawberry Kiwi Quencher. 80

Tropical Turmeric Twist. 80

Raspberry Coconut Dream 81

Spinach and Apple Detox 81

Mint Chocolate Chip Delight. 82

Chia Berry Blast 82

Vanilla Fig Smoothie 83

Watermelon Cucumber Cooler. 83

DESSERTS 85

Banana-Oatmeal Cookies 85

Chocolate Protein Balls. 85

Avocado Chocolate Brownies. 86

Lemon Poppy Seed Cake 86

Vanilla Almond Biscotti. 87

Strawberry Yogurt Cake. 88

Mango and Lime Sorbet Bars 88

Almond and Date Energy Bites. 89

Blueberry Oatmeal Cookies 89

Cinnamon Raisin Scones 90

Cherry Almond Muffins 90

Carrot Cake Bars 91

Gingerbread Cookies. 92

Baked Apricots with Almond Crumble. 92

Cranberry Orange Scones 93

Coconut Macaroons 93

28-DAY MEAL PLAN 95
CONCLUSION 97

INTRODUCTION

Thriving Without a Gallbladder: Your Guide to Life Post-Surgery

Living without a gallbladder is a reality for many individuals who have undergone cholecystectomy, the surgical removal of the gallbladder. While this procedure is often necessary to alleviate pain and health issues, it can raise questions about diet and digestion.

Understanding Life After Gallbladder Removal

The gallbladder plays a crucial role in digestion by storing and releasing bile, which helps break down fats in our foods. When you remove it, the body can still digest fats, but the process may be altered. As a result, some individuals experience digestive discomfort, particularly after consuming fatty or greasy foods.

Lifestyle Considerations

Living well without a gallbladder isn't just about diet but holistic health. Consider these lifestyle factors:

1. **Regular exercise:** Physical activity can aid digestion, promote well-being, and help manage weight.
2. **Manage Stress:** High-stress levels can affect digestion. Incorporate stress management techniques like meditation, yoga, or deep breathing into your routine.
3. **Listen to Your Body:** How your body responds to different foods and situations. Your body is your best guide.
4. **Regular Check-Ups:** Schedule regular check-ups with your healthcare provider to monitor your health and discuss any concerns or changes in your digestion.
5. **Seek Support:** If you're struggling with dietary changes or digestive issues, consider consulting a registered dietitian or nutritionist who can provide personalized guidance.

Nurturing Your Gallbladder Health: Tips for Optimal Digestion

While gallbladder removal is a standard procedure, many individuals seek ways to enhance their digestion and overall well-being in its absence. Here are some tips and strategies to support your gallbladder health and improve digestive comfort, even after gallbladder surgery.

- **Embrace a Balanced Diet** Maintaining a well-balanced diet is crucial for overall digestive health. Focus on including a variety of whole foods such as fruits, vegetables, lean proteins, whole grains, and healthy fats in your meals. A balanced diet provides essential nutrients and supports overall digestion.

- **Prioritize Fiber** Fiber is a digestive powerhouse. It aids in bowel regularity and prevents constipation. Incorporate high-fiber foods like leafy greens, whole grains, legumes, and fruits into your diet to support healthy digestion.

- **Stay Hydrated** Adequate hydration is essential for digestion. Water helps break down food, move it through the digestive tract, and prevent constipation. Aim to drink plenty of water throughout the day to support smooth digestion.

- **Chew Your Food Thoroughly** Digestion begins in the mouth. Chewing your food thoroughly not only aids in breaking down food but also helps reduce the workload on your digestive system. Take your time with each bite, savoring the flavors and textures.

- **Eat Smaller, More Frequent Meals** Instead of three large meals, consider eating smaller, more frequent meals throughout the day. Small portions can help prevent overloading your digestive system and reduce the likelihood of discomfort.

- **Choose Lean Proteins** Opt for lean protein sources like poultry, fish, tofu, and legumes. These are easier to digest than fatty cuts of meat, which can be more challenging for your digestive system to process.

- **Incorporate Healthy Fats** While you may need to watch your fat intake, including healthy fats in your diet is essential. Olive oil, avocados, nuts, and seeds provide essential fatty acids and can support gallbladder health.

- **Mindful Eating Practices** Practice mindful eating by savoring your meals and paying attention to hunger and fullness cues. Avoid eating too quickly or while distracted, leading to overeating and digestive discomfort.

- **Limit Trigger Foods** Certain foods may trigger

digestive discomfort for some individuals. Please keep track of any specific foods that seem to cause issues and consider reducing or eliminating them from your diet.

- **Herbal Support** Some herbs, such as ginger and peppermint, have been known to support digestion. Consider incorporating these into your meals or enjoying them as teas to soothe digestive discomfort.

- **Manage Stress** Stress can have a significant impact on digestion. Use stress-reduction practices like yoga, meditation, or deep breathing exercises to support your overall well-being and digestion.

- **Consult a Healthcare Provider** If you continue to experience digestive issues or discomfort after gallbladder surgery, consult a healthcare provider. They can offer guidance, recommend dietary adjustments, or explore other treatment options to address your needs.

Strategies for Reducing Gallbladder Attacks and Managing Pain

Living without a gallbladder doesn't mean enduring frequent gallbladder attacks and persistent discomfort. Let's explore practical ideas for reducing the likelihood of gallbladder attacks and strategies to ease the pain when they occur, helping you find comfort and relief.

1. **Follow a Low-Fat Diet** A low-fat diet remains a cornerstone of gallbladder health. Limit your high-fat and fried food intake, as these can trigger attacks. Instead, focus on lean proteins, whole grains, and healthy fats in moderation.

2. **Gradually Reintroduce Fats** After gallbladder surgery, it's essential to reintroduce fats slowly into your diet. Start with small amounts of healthy fats like olive oil or avocados and gradually increase as your body adapts.

3. **Include Fiber-Rich Foods** Fiber-rich foods, such as fruits, vegetables, and whole grains, can aid digestion and prevent constipation, which can contribute to gallstone formation and discomfort.

4. **Stay Hydrated** Adequate hydration is vital for overall health and can help prevent gallstone formation. Drink plenty of water throughout the day to support your digestive system.

5. **Ginger for Nausea** If nausea accompanies a gallbladder attack, ginger can help soothe your stomach. Try ginger tea or ginger candies to alleviate nausea symptoms.

6. **Over-the-Counter Pain Relief** Over-the-counter pain relievers, such as ibuprofen or acetaminophen, can temporarily relieve gallbladder pain. Always follow the recommended dosage and consult your healthcare provider if the pain persists.

7. **Heat Therapy** Applying a warm compress or heating pad to the upper right abdomen where the gallbladder used to be can help alleviate pain and discomfort during an attack.

8. **Avoid Tight Clothing** Wearing tight clothing, especially around the waist, can pressure the abdomen and exacerbate gallbladder pain. Opt for loose-fitting attire during episodes of discomfort.

9. **Relaxation Techniques** Stress can trigger or worsen gallbladder attacks. Engage in relaxation techniques such as deep breathing exercises, meditation, or gentle yoga to reduce stress and promote pain relief.

10. **Consult with a Healthcare Provider** If gallbladder attacks are severe, frequent, or accompanied by concerning symptoms, it's crucial to consult with a healthcare provider. They can provide a tailored treatment plan, including medication or further interventions if necessary.

Managing gallbladder attacks and the associated pain requires a multifaceted approach encompassing dietary adjustments, lifestyle changes, and stress management. By incorporating these strategies and actively engaging in your health and well-being, you can reduce the frequency and severity of gallbladder attacks, ultimately leading to a more comfortable and enjoyable post-gallbladder life. Remember that everyone's experience is unique, so it's essential to consult with a healthcare provider for personalized guidance and treatment options when needed.

Natural Remedies for Promoting Digestive Wellness After Gallbladder Removal

In addition to dietary changes, several safe and natural remedies can contribute to your gallbladder's well-being and overall digestive system. These remedies help maintain balance, reduce discomfort, and promote digestive health. Let's explore these holistic approaches to support your digestive system.

- **Milk Thistle** Milk thistle is renowned for its potential to promote liver health. It contains an active compound called silymarin, which may help protect liver cells and support bile production. Consult with a healthcare provider before adding milk thistle supplements to your regimen.

- **Dandelion Root** Dandelion root is another herb that supports liver and gallbladder health. It may enhance bile flow and promote overall digestive function. You can brew dandelion root tea or find it in supplement form.

- **Artichoke Leaf** Artichoke leaf extract has been shown to stimulate bile production and improve digestion. It can be a valuable addition to your supplements under the guidance of a healthcare provider.

- **Turmeric and Curcumin** With its active compound, curcumin, turmeric offers anti-inflammatory properties and may aid digestion. Incorporate turmeric into your cooking or discuss curcumin supplements with your healthcare provider.

- **Marshmallow Root** Marshmallow root can help soothe the digestive tract, reducing irritation and inflammation. It's available in various forms, including teas and supplements, and may relieve indigestion.

- **Slippery Elm** Slippery elm is known for its ability to coat and soothe the digestive tract. It can be beneficial for addressing issues like heartburn and indigestion. Slippery elm supplements or teas are available.

- **Aloe Vera** Aloe vera is soothing for the skin and can support digestive health. Pure, food-grade aloe vera juice may help reduce inflammation and discomfort.

- **Probiotics** Probiotics are beneficial bacteria that foster a healthy gut microbiome. Maintaining a balanced gut environment is crucial for overall digestion. Consult with a healthcare provider to find a probiotic that suits your needs.

- **Digestive Enzymes** Digestive enzyme supplements can aid in the breakdown of foods, making them easier for your digestive system to handle. These supplements can be beneficial if you experience difficulties digesting certain foods.

- **Ginger** Ginger famous for its anti-inflammatory and digestive properties. Incorporate fresh ginger into your meals, brew ginger tea, or enjoy ginger supplements to support digestive comfort.

- **Fennel Seeds** Chewing fennel seeds after meals can help alleviate bloating and gas. Fennel tea is another delightful option to promote digestive ease.

- **Lemon Water** Starting your day with warm lemon water can stimulate the liver and encourage bile production, potentially aiding fat and overall digestion.

These natural remedies offer valuable support for gallbladder and digestive health. However, it's essential to consult with a healthcare provider before introducing any new supplements or herbs into your routine, especially if you have underlying health conditions or take medications. Combining dietary changes with these natural remedies can foster a harmonious relationship with your digestive system, leading to greater comfort and well-being in your post-gallbladder life.

Navigating Life After Gallbladder Surgery: A Comprehensive Guide to Health and Well-being

Gallbladder surgery, or cholecystectomy, is a significant medical procedure that can relieve gallstones and related health issues. While the surgical removal of the gallbladder is standard, it marks a pivotal moment in your digestive health journey. In this chapter, we'll delve into the critical aspects of gallbladder surgery and how to lead a healthy and fulfilling life once your gallbladder is no longer a part of your digestive system.

Understanding Gallbladder Surgery

Gallbladder surgery involves the removal of the gallbladder—a small organ located beneath the liver. This surgery is typically performed to alleviate gallstones, which can cause intense pain and other complications. Two primary types of cholecystectomy exist:

1. **Laparoscopic Cholecystectomy:** In this minimally invasive procedure, small incisions are made, and a laparoscope removes the gallbladder. Recovery time is generally shorter compared to open surgery.

2. **Open Cholecystectomy:** This procedure involves a larger incision in the abdomen to remove the gallbladder. It's reserved for

specific cases where laparoscopic surgery isn't suitable.

Life After Gallbladder Surgery

Living healthily after gallbladder surgery requires a few adjustments to your diet and lifestyle. Here's what you need to know:

1. **Dietary Changes:** Without a gallbladder, your body still produces bile, but it's no longer stored for release when you eat. Bile continuously trickles into your digestive tract, making it harder for your body to process large amounts of fat simultaneously. Adjust your diet by:

   - Gradually reintroducing fats, starting with healthy options like olive oil.
   - Eating smaller, more frequent meals to prevent overloading your digestive system.
   - Focusing on lean proteins, whole grains, and fiber-rich foods.
   - Monitoring your body's response to different foods and identifying any trigger foods that may cause discomfort.

2. **Mindful Eating:** Practice mindful eating by savoring your meals, chewing your food thoroughly, and paying attention to your body's hunger and fullness cues. Avoid eating too quickly or while distracted, leading to overeating and digestive discomfort.

3. **Stress Management:** High-stress levels can negatively impact digestion. Use stress-reduction practices like meditation, yoga, or deep breathing exercises to support your overall well-being and digestion.

4. **Regular Check-Ups:** Schedule regular check-ups with your healthcare provider to monitor your health, discuss any concerns, and adjust your post-surgery plan if needed.

Gallbladder surgery is a significant step toward relieving gallstone-related discomfort. Still, it marks the beginning of a new chapter in your digestive health journey. You can lead a fulfilling and healthy life without your gallbladder by making thoughtful dietary choices, staying attuned to your body's signals, and adopting a balanced lifestyle. Everyone's experience is unique, so consult with healthcare professionals when necessary to ensure your well-being as you embark on this post-surgery phase of your life.

Foods to Embrace and Foods to Avoid After Gallbladder Removal

Your diet plays a pivotal role in post-gallbladder surgery life. Knowing which foods to include and which to avoid is vital to promoting digestive comfort and overall well-being. This chapter will provide a comprehensive guide to help you make informed dietary choices on your journey toward a healthier and happier post-gallbladder life.

Foods to Embrace: Supporting Digestive Comfort

- **Lean Proteins:** Prioritize lean protein sources, such as skinless poultry, fish, tofu, and legumes. These are easier for your digestive system to handle than fatty cuts of meat.
- **Whole Grains:** Whole grains like oats, brown rice, quinoa, and whole wheat bread provide Fiber to support digestion and prevent constipation.
- **Fruits:** Opt for low-acid fruits like apples, pears, and berries. These are gentle on your stomach and provide essential vitamins and Fiber.
- **Vegetables:** Non-cruciferous vegetables like leafy greens, carrots, and zucchini are generally well-tolerated and rich in nutrients.
- **Healthy Fats:** While limiting overall fat intake, include healthy fats like olive oil, avocados, nuts, and seeds in moderation. These provide essential fatty acids without overwhelming your digestion.
- **Low-Fat Dairy:** If you tolerate dairy well, choose low-fat or fat-free options like yogurt or skim milk. Dairy alternatives like almond or soy milk can also be suitable.
- **Herbs and Spices:** Flavor your dishes with herbs and spices like ginger, turmeric, mint, and basil. These can enhance taste without adding unnecessary fat.
- **Probiotic Foods:** Incorporate probiotic-rich foods like yogurt with live cultures, kefir, and fermented vegetables to support a healthy gut microbiome and overall digestion.
- **Foods to Limit or Avoid:** Potential Digestive Triggers
- **High-Fat Foods:** Steer clear of high-fat and fried foods, as they can be challenging to digest without a gallbladder.
- **Greasy Foods:** Foods cooked in heavy oils or butter can trigger digestive discomfort. Opt for

cooking methods like grilling, steaming, or baking instead.

- **Spicy Foods:** Spicy dishes may irritate your digestive tract. If you enjoy spices, use them in moderation and pay attention to how your body responds.

- **Processed Foods:** Highly processed foods often contain hidden fats and additives that can be harsh on digestion. Opt for whole, unprocessed options whenever possible.

- **Excessive Dairy:** While some individuals tolerate dairy well, it can be problematic for others. Monitor your body's response to dairy and choose low-fat or dairy alternatives.

- **High-Acidity Foods:** Acidic foods like citrus fruits, tomatoes, and vinegar may trigger discomfort in some individuals. Adjust your consumption based on your tolerance.

- **Carbonated Beverages:** Carbonated drinks can lead to gas and bloating. Consider reducing or eliminating them from your diet.

- **Alcohol:** Alcohol can be taxing on the liver and digestive system. Consume alcohol in moderation and pay attention to how it affects you.

Navigating your diet after gallbladder removal is about finding a balance that suits your unique needs and preferences. You can promote digestive comfort and overall health by focusing on lean proteins, whole grains, low-acid fruits, and well-tolerated vegetables, avoiding high-fat and greasy foods. Remember that your body's response to specific foods may vary, so listen to its signals and adjust your diet accordingly. You can embrace a nourishing and satisfying post-gallbladder life with mindful dietary choices.

Embracing the Benefits of a Thoughtful Diet After Gallbladder Removal

A well-considered diet after gallbladder removal can bring numerous benefits beyond just alleviating discomfort. Let's explore the advantages of making informed dietary choices in your post-gallbladder life, highlighting how these can contribute to your overall well-being.

1. **Improved Digestive Comfort** One of the most significant benefits of a mindful post-gallbladder diet is improved digestive comfort. Avoiding or limiting foods that can trigger discomfort can significantly reduce the likelihood of digestive issues such as bloating, gas, and diarrhea. Reducing triggering food can lead to a more comfortable and pain-free existence.

2. **Enhanced Nutrient Absorption** A well-balanced diet that includes a variety of nutrient-rich foods supports optimal nutrient absorption. Without a gallbladder, your body may require extra assistance breaking down and absorbing essential nutrients, such as fat-soluble vitamins (A, D, E, and K). By choosing nutrient-dense foods, you can ensure your body receives the vital nutrients it needs to thrive.

3. **Weight Management** A thoughtful diet can also help with weight management. You can maintain a balanced weight by focusing on lean proteins, whole grains, and fiber-rich foods. Including whole food in your ration, in turn, reduces the risk of obesity-related health issues and supports your overall health and well-being.

4. **Stable Blood Sugar Levels** A diet prioritizing complex carbohydrates and fiber-rich foods can help stabilize blood sugar levels. This can be particularly beneficial for individuals with diabetes or those at risk of developing the condition, contributing to better long-term health outcomes.

5. **Support for the Liver** The liver plays a crucial role in digestion and overall health. A diet that minimizes the consumption of high-fat and greasy foods can ease the workload on your liver. Additionally, foods like artichoke leaf extract and milk thistle may support liver health and bile production.

6. **Balanced Gut Microbiome** Consuming probiotic-rich foods like yogurt and kefir can promote a healthy gut microbiome. A balanced gut environment is essential for proper digestion and overall well-being. A diet that includes these foods can contribute to a thriving gut microbiota.

7. **Reduced Risk of Gallstone Formation** Adopting a low-fat diet and avoiding trigger foods may reduce the risk of forming new gallstones without a gallbladder. Maintaining a gallstone-free status can minimize the potential for future gallstone-related complications.

8. **Holistic Well-Being** A well-considered diet is a cornerstone of holistic well-being. It's not just about physical health; it's also about nourishing

your body, fostering mental clarity, and promoting emotional balance. When you feel good physically, it positively impacts all aspects of your life.

The benefits of a thoughtful diet after gallbladder removal extend far beyond digestive comfort. By making informed dietary choices that support your overall health, you can enhance nutrient absorption, manage your weight, stabilize blood sugar levels, and reduce the risk of future gallstone formation. Your diet plays a vital role in your holistic well-being, and embracing a nourishing approach to post-gallbladder life can lead to a healthier, happier, and more vibrant existence.

Common Questions and Expert Answers for Your Post-Gallbladder Diet Journey

As you embark on your post-gallbladder diet journey, you may have numerous questions and concerns. In this chapter, we'll address some of the most common queries individuals have after gallbladder removal, providing expert answers to help you navigate this new phase of your digestive health.

Q1: Can I ever eat fatty foods again after gallbladder surgery?

A1: You can eventually reintroduce moderate amounts of healthy fats into your diet. After gallbladder surgery, it's essential to reintroduce fats and monitor your body's response gradually. Start with healthy options like olive oil, avocados, and fatty fish, and slowly increase your fat intake. Listen to your body, as everyone's tolerance for fats can vary.

Q2: Are there any specific foods I should avoid indefinitely?

A2: While you can reintroduce most foods into your diet, it's wise to avoid or limit high-fat, greasy, and spicy foods indefinitely. These can be challenging to digest without a gallbladder and may trigger discomfort. Monitor your response to foods like dairy, high-acid fruits, and carbonated beverages, and adjust your consumption based on your tolerance.

Q3: Will I need to take digestive supplements after gallbladder removal?

A3: Some individuals find digestive enzyme supplements helpful, especially when consuming higher-fat meals. These supplements can assist in breaking down fats, making digestion more comfortable. Probiotics may also be beneficial for maintaining a healthy gut microbiome and overall digestive health. Consult your healthcare provider to determine if these supplements are right for you.

Q4: Can I still enjoy spicy foods and alcohol occasionally?

A4: Spicy foods and alcohol can irritate the digestive tract and may trigger discomfort. However, some individuals tolerate them in moderation. If you enjoy these items, consume them sparingly and pay attention to how your body responds. It's crucial to listen to your body's signals and adjust your diet accordingly.

Q5: How can I manage weight after gallbladder surgery?

A5: Maintaining a balanced diet emphasizing lean proteins, whole grains, and fiber-rich foods can help manage weight. Portion control and mindful eating practices are also essential. Regular physical activity, tailored to your fitness level, can further support weight management and overall well-being.

Q6: Can I ever enjoy rich, indulgent meals again?

A6: While you may need to be mindful of your fat intake, you can still enjoy occasional indulgent meals. Consider reserving such meals for special occasions and balancing them with lighter, low-fat options in your regular diet. Moderation is vital to enjoying rich foods without discomfort.

Q7: How long does it take to adapt to a post-gallbladder diet?

A7: Adapting to a post-gallbladder diet varies from person to person. Some individuals adjust quickly, while others may take several months to fine-tune their dietary choices. Patience is essential. Keep a food diary to track what works for you, consult with healthcare professionals as needed, and make gradual adjustments over time.

Q8: Are there any long-term health concerns I should be aware of?

A8: In the absence of your gallbladder, you should be mindful of your fat intake, monitor your tolerance for specific foods, and prioritize a well-balanced diet. Long-term health concerns can include weight management, the risk of gallstone formation, and overall digestive health. Regular check-ups with your healthcare provider can help address any potential issues proactively.

As you embark on your post-gallbladder diet journey, remember that you're not alone in your quest for digestive comfort and well-being. Typical questions addressed in this chapter are part of the learning process. By seeking expert answers, making informed dietary choices, and listening to your body, you can confidently navigate this new phase of your digestive health and embrace a vibrant, post-gallbladder life.

The Non-Gallbladder Diet Essentials: Serving Size Guidelines and Meal Planning Principles

Understanding the basics of a non-gallbladder diet, including portion sizes and meal planning principles, is crucial for maintaining digestive comfort and overall well-being. We'll provide essential information to help you successfully navigate your post-gallbladder diet.

Serving Size Guidelines

Proper portion control is critical to preventing digestive discomfort and managing fat intake. Here are some serving size guidelines to keep in mind:

1. **Lean Proteins:** Aim for 3-4 ounces (85-113 grams) of lean protein per meal. Proteins can include skinless poultry, fish, tofu, or legumes. Remember that lean cuts of meat contain less fat.

2. **Healthy Fats:** When incorporating healthy fats like olive oil or avocado into your meals, limit the portion to 1-2 tablespoons per serving. This amount provides essential fatty acids without overwhelming your digestion.

3. **Whole Grains:** Enjoy ½ to 1 cup (90-180 grams) of cooked whole grains like brown rice, quinoa, or whole wheat pasta. These grains are rich in Fiber and nutrients, supporting healthy digestion.

4. **Fruits:** Consume one serving of low-acid fruits per meal, typically a small apple, a pear, or a handful of berries. These fruits are gentle on the stomach and provide essential vitamins.

5. **Non-Cruciferous Vegetables:** Include 1-2 servings of non-cruciferous vegetables, such as leafy greens, carrots, or zucchini, in each meal. These vegetables are generally well-tolerated and nutrient-rich.

6. **Dairy or Dairy Alternatives:** If you tolerate dairy well, choose ½ to 1 cup (120-240 milliliters) of low-fat yogurt or a dairy alternative like almond milk. Dairy options with live cultures are ideal for supporting gut health.

7. **Herbs and Spices:** When using herbs and spices to flavor your dishes, a pinch or a teaspoon is usually sufficient. Experiment to find the right balance for your palate.

General Meal Planning Principles

Creating well-balanced, digestive-friendly meals involves more than portion sizes. Here are some general meal-planning principles to keep in mind:

Consistent Meal Timing: Aim to eat meals regularly throughout the day. Eating smaller, more frequent meals can prevent overloading your digestive system.

1. **Balanced Macros:** Each meal should ideally balance carbohydrates, proteins, and fats. This balance helps stabilize blood sugar levels and supports overall digestion.

2. **Fiber-Rich Foods:** Incorporate fiber-rich foods like fruits, vegetables, and whole grains into your meals. Fiber aids digestion and prevents constipation.

3. **Mindful Eating:** Practice mindful eating by savoring your meals, chewing thoroughly, and paying attention to your body's hunger and fullness cues. Avoid eating too quickly or while distracted..

4. **Supplements:** Consider discussing the use of digestive enzyme supplements and probiotics with your healthcare provider to support digestion and gut health.

Following serving size guidelines and adhering to these meal planning principles, you can craft well-balanced and digestive-friendly meals that support your overall well-being. Remember that your body's response to food may vary, so listening to its signals and adjusting your diet as needed is essential. With a thoughtful and informed approach to meal planning, you can confidently navigate your non-gallbladder diet and embrace a nourishing post-gallbladder life.

Breakfast

Creamy Oatmeal with Fresh Berries

Serving: 4 | Prep time: 10 minutes | Cook time: 15 minutes

Ingredients:

- 12 oz (340 g) rolled oats
- 32 oz (946 ml) almond milk
- 4 oz (113 g) fresh mixed berries (strawberries, blueberries, raspberries)
- 2 oz (57 g) honey
- 2 oz (57 g) plain Greek yogurt
- 1 tsp vanilla extract
- 1 tsp ground cinnamon
- 1 oz (28 g) chopped almonds
- 1 oz (28 g) ground flaxseed
- Fresh mint leaves for garnish

Directions:

1. In a medium saucepan, bring the almond milk to a gentle simmer over medium heat.
2. Stir in the rolled oats and reduce the heat to low. Cook for about 10-15 minutes, stirring occasionally, until the oats have absorbed most of the liquid and reached your desired creamy consistency.
3. While the oatmeal is cooking, in a small bowl, mix together the honey, vanilla extract, and Greek yogurt until well combined.
4. Once the oatmeal is ready, remove it from heat and stir in the honey and yogurt mixture, ground cinnamon, and half of the fresh berries.
5. Divide the creamy oatmeal among four serving bowls. Top each serving with the remaining fresh berries, chopped almonds, and ground flaxseed.
6. Garnish with fresh mint leaves for a burst of color and flavor.

Useful Tip: To make this oatmeal even creamier, you can substitute some of the almond milk with unsweetened coconut milk or cashew milk for a richer texture.

Nutritional Values: Calories: 340 kcal | Fat: 10 g | Protein: 10 g | Carbs: 57 g | Net carbs: 47 g | Fiber: 10 g | Cholesterol: 0 mg | Sodium: 90 mg | Potassium: 375 mg

Scrambled Eggs with Spinach and Feta

Serving: 4 | Prep time: 10 minutes | Cook time: 10 minutes

Ingredients:

- 8 large eggs
- 4 oz (113 g) fresh spinach, chopped
- 4 oz (113 g) crumbled feta cheese
- 2 oz (57 g) unsalted butter
- 1 oz (28 g) chopped green onions
- 1/2 tsp garlic powder
- Salt and pepper to taste

Directions:

1. Crack the eggs into a bowl and whisk them until well beaten.
2. In a large non-stick skillet over medium-low heat, melt the butter.
3. Add the chopped spinach and green onions to the skillet and sauté for about 2-3 minutes until the spinach wilts.
4. Pour the beaten eggs over the spinach and stir gently with a wooden spoon.
5. As the eggs start to set, sprinkle in the crumbled feta cheese, garlic powder, salt, and pepper. Continue to gently stir until the eggs are fully cooked but still creamy, about 5-7 minutes.
6. Once the eggs reach your desired consistency, remove the skillet from heat.

Useful Tip: For a creamier texture, you can add a splash of unsweetened almond milk to the beaten eggs before cooking.

Nutritional Values: Calories: 240 kcal | Fat: 18 g | Protein: 15 g | Carbs: 4 g | Net carbs: 2 g | Fiber: 2 g | Cholesterol: 350 mg | Sodium: 360 mg | Potassium: 360 mg

Banana Walnut Pancakes

Serving: 4 | Prep time: 15 minutes | Cook time: 10 minutes

Ingredients:

- 2 ripe bananas, mashed (about 6 oz or 170 g)
- 4 large eggs
- 2 oz (57 g) almond flour
- 2 oz (57 g) chopped walnuts
- 1 oz (28 g) unsalted butter, melted
- 1 tsp baking powder
- 1 tsp ground cinnamon
- 1/2 tsp vanilla extract
- Pinch of salt
- Cooking spray

Directions:

1. In a mixing bowl, combine the mashed bananas, eggs, melted butter, and vanilla extract.
2. In a separate bowl, mix the almond flour, baking powder, ground cinnamon, and a pinch of salt.
3. Gradually add the dry ingredients to the banana mixture, stirring until well combined.
4. Gently fold in the chopped walnuts, ensuring they are evenly distributed throughout the batter.
5. Preheat a non-stick skillet or griddle over medium-low heat. Lightly grease it with a small amount of butter or cooking spray.
6. Pour a ladleful of pancake batter onto the skillet for each pancake and spread it into a circular shape.
7. Cook the pancakes for about 2-3 minutes on each side, or until they are golden brown and cooked through.

Useful Tip: If you prefer a sweeter flavor without adding sugar, you can drizzle a small amount of honey or maple syrup over the pancakes before serving.

Nutritional Values: Calories: 290 kcal | Fat: 21 g | Protein: 9 g | Carbs: 18 g | Net carbs: 12 g | Fiber: 6 g | Cholesterol: 200 mg | Sodium: 170 mg | Potassium: 310 mg

Greek Yogurt Parfait

Serving: 4 | Prep time: 10 minutes | Cook time: 0 minutes

Ingredients:

- 16 oz (454 g) plain Greek yogurt
- 8 oz (227 g) mixed berries (strawberries, blueberries, raspberries)
- 2 oz (57 g) chopped almonds
- 2 oz (57 g) honey
- 1 oz (28 g) unsweetened coconut flakes
- 1 tsp vanilla extract
- 1 tsp ground cinnamon

Directions:

1. In a bowl, combine the plain Greek yogurt and vanilla extract, and mix until smooth.
2. In serving glasses or bowls, start with a layer of the Greek yogurt mixture.
3. Add a layer of mixed berries on top of the yogurt.
4. Sprinkle a layer of chopped almonds and unsweetened coconut flakes over the berries.
5. Drizzle a bit of honey over the almond and coconut layer.
6. Repeat the layers until the glasses are filled, finishing with a dollop of Greek yogurt on top.
7. Sprinkle a pinch of ground cinnamon over each parfait for added flavor.

Useful Tip: Customize your parfaits by adding other gallbladder-friendly ingredients like chia seeds, ground flaxseed, or a dash of lemon zest for a refreshing twist.

Nutritional Values: Calories: 260 kcal | Fat: 13 g | Protein: 17 g | Carbs: 26 g | Net carbs: 18 g | Fiber: 8 g | Cholesterol: 10 mg | Sodium: 40 mg | Potassium: 330 mg

Apple Cinnamon Quinoa Porridge

Serving: 4 | Prep time: 10 minutes | Cook time: 20 minutes

Ingredients:

- 8 oz (227 g) quinoa, rinsed and drained
- 32 oz (946 ml) unsweetened almond milk
- 2 medium apples, peeled, cored, and diced (about 12 oz or 340 g)
- 2 oz (57 g) chopped walnuts
- 2 oz (57 g) honey
- 1 tsp ground cinnamon
- 1/2 tsp vanilla extract
- Pinch of salt

Directions:

1. In a medium saucepan, combine the rinsed quinoa and almond milk. Bring it to a boil over medium-high heat.
2. Once boiling, reduce the heat to low, cover, and let it simmer for 15-20 minutes, or until the quinoa is tender and most of the liquid is absorbed.
3. While the quinoa is cooking, in a separate skillet, sauté the diced apples over medium heat with a pinch of salt, honey, and ground cinnamon until they become soft and slightly caramelized, about 5-7 minutes.
4. When the quinoa is ready, remove it from heat and stir in the vanilla extract.
5. Divide the cooked quinoa among serving bowls.
6. Top each bowl with the sautéed apples and chopped walnuts.
7. Drizzle a touch of honey over the top for added sweetness and garnish with an extra sprinkle of ground cinnamon if desired.

Useful Tip: For added creaminess, mix a spoonful of unsweetened Greek yogurt into the porridge just before serving.

Nutritional Values: Calories: 330 kcal | Fat: 11 g | Protein: 7 g | Carbs: 53 g | Net carbs: 39 g | Fiber: 14 g | Cholesterol: 0 mg | Sodium: 180 mg | Potassium: 490 mg

Avocado Toast with Poached Eggs

Serving: 4 | Prep time: 15 minutes | Cook time: 10 minutes

Ingredients:

- 8 slices of whole-grain bread (about 16 oz or 454 g)
- 4 ripe avocados (about 16 oz or 454 g)
- 4 large eggs
- oz (28 g) fresh spinach leaves
- 2 oz (57 g) cherry tomatoes, halved
- 1 oz (28 g) feta cheese, crumbled
- 1 tsp olive oil
- 1 tsp lemon juice
- 1 tsp white vinegar
- Salt and pepper to taste

Directions:

1. Begin by toasting the whole-grain bread until it's crisp and golden brown.
2. While the bread is toasting, halve the avocados, remove the pits, and scoop the flesh into a bowl. Mash the avocado with a fork, leaving it slightly chunky.
3. In a separate saucepan, bring water to a gentle simmer, then add a dash of white vinegar.
4. Carefully crack each egg into a small cup or ramekin. Create a gentle whirlpool in the simmering water using a spoon and slide the eggs one by one into the swirling water. Poach for about 3-4 minutes until the whites are set but the yolks are still runny.
5. While the eggs are poaching, toss the fresh spinach leaves with olive oil, lemon juice, salt, and pepper in a bowl.
6. Spread the mashed avocado evenly on each slice of toasted bread.
7. Place the dressed spinach on top of the avocado, followed by the poached eggs.
8. Scatter halved cherry tomatoes and crumbled feta cheese over the poached eggs.

Useful Tip: To make poaching eggs easier, crack each egg into a fine-mesh strainer over a bowl to drain off excess liquid before transferring it to the simmering water.

Nutritional Values: Calories: 320 kcal | Fat: 18 g | Protein: 13 g | Carbs: 30 g | Net carbs: 20 g | Fiber: 10 g | Cholesterol: 185 mg | Sodium: 360 mg | Potassium: 990 mg

Sweet Potato Hash with Turkey Sausage

Serving: 4 | Prep time: 15 minutes | Cook time: 25 minutes

Ingredients:

- 16 oz (454 g) sweet potatoes, peeled and diced
- 12 oz (340 g) lean turkey sausage, crumbled
- 8 oz (227 g) bell peppers, diced
- 4 oz (113 g) red onion, finely chopped
- 2 oz (57 g) baby spinach
- 1 oz (28 g) olive oil
- 1 tsp smoked paprika
- 1/2 tsp garlic powder
- Salt and pepper to taste
- Fresh parsley for garnish

Directions:

1. Heat the olive oil in a large skillet over medium heat.
2. Add the diced sweet potatoes to the skillet and cook for about 10-12 minutes, stirring occasionally, until they are tender and slightly browned.
3. In the same skillet, push the sweet potatoes to one side and add the crumbled turkey sausage. Cook it until it's no longer pink, breaking it up with a spatula as it cooks.
4. Stir in the diced bell peppers and red onion, and cook for an additional 5-7 minutes, until the vegetables are tender.
5. Add the smoked paprika, garlic powder, salt, and pepper to the skillet. Stir well to evenly coat the ingredients with the spices.
6. Finally, add the baby spinach to the skillet and cook for 2-3 minutes until it wilts and combines with the rest of the ingredients.
7. Serve the sweet potato hash hot, garnished with a sprinkle of fresh parsley if desired.

Useful Tip: To make this dish extra flavorful, consider adding a dash of hot sauce or a pinch of crushed red pepper flakes for a spicy kick.

Nutritional Values: Calories: 320 kcal | Fat: 18 g | Protein: 15 g | Carbs: 25 g | Net carbs: 18 g | Fiber: 7 g | Cholesterol: 45 mg | Sodium: 540 mg | Potassium: 630 mg

Blueberry Chia Pudding

Serving: 4 | Prep time: 10 minutes | Cook time: 0 minutes

Ingredients:

- 4 oz (113 g) fresh blueberries
- 2 oz (57 g) chia seeds
- 16 oz (473 ml) unsweetened almond milk
- 2 oz (57 g) honey
- 1 tsp vanilla extract
- 1 oz (28 g) unsweetened coconut flakes
- 1 oz (28 g) sliced almonds

Directions:

1. In a blender, combine the fresh blueberries, almond milk, honey, and vanilla extract. Blend until smooth.
2. In a mixing bowl, whisk together the chia seeds and the blended blueberry mixture.
3. Cover the bowl and refrigerate for at least 2 hours, or until the chia seeds have absorbed the liquid and the mixture has thickened to a pudding-like consistency. Stir occasionally during this time to prevent clumping.
4. When the chia pudding is ready, divide it among serving glasses or bowls.
5. Top each serving with a handful of fresh blueberries, unsweetened coconut flakes, and sliced almonds for added texture and flavor.

Useful Tip: To enhance the flavor and nutritional profile, you can add a pinch of ground cinnamon or a drizzle of almond butter before serving.

Nutritional Values: Calories: 250 kcal | Fat: 12 g | Protein: 5 g | Carbs: 30 g | Net carbs: 20 g | Fiber: 10 g | Cholesterol: 0 mg | Sodium: 60 mg | Potassium: 280 mg

Spinach and Mushroom Breakfast Burrito

Serving: 4 | Prep time: 15 minutes | Cook time: 15 minutes

Ingredients:

- 8 large eggs
- 8 oz (227 g) fresh spinach
- 8 oz (227 g) mushrooms, sliced
- 4 oz (113 g) diced red bell pepper
- 4 oz (113 g) diced red onion
- 4 oz (113 g) feta cheese, crumbled
- 4 whole-grain tortillas
- 2 oz (57 g) olive oil
- 1 tsp garlic powder
- Salt and pepper to taste

Directions:

1. In a large skillet, heat the olive oil over medium-high heat.
2. Add the sliced mushrooms and diced red onion to the skillet. Sauté for about 5 minutes until the mushrooms become golden brown and the onions are translucent.
3. Add the diced red bell pepper and fresh spinach to the skillet. Continue to cook for another 2-3 minutes until the spinach wilts and the pepper softens.
4. In a separate bowl, whisk together the eggs, garlic powder, salt, and pepper.
5. Pour the egg mixture into the skillet with the sautéed vegetables. Cook, stirring occasionally, until the eggs are fully scrambled and cooked through, about 3-5 minutes.
6. Warm the whole-grain tortillas in a dry skillet for about 10 seconds on each side or microwave them for a few seconds to make them pliable.
7. Divide the scrambled egg mixture evenly among the tortillas.
8. Sprinkle crumbled feta cheese over the eggs in each tortilla.
9. Roll up the tortillas, folding in the sides as you go to create burritos.

Useful Tip: For a spicier kick, you can add a dash of hot sauce or sprinkle red pepper flakes into the scrambled egg mixture before cooking.

Nutritional Values: Calories: 330 kcal | Fat: 20 g | Protein: 16 g | Carbs: 23 g | Net carbs: 16 g | Fiber: 7 g | Cholesterol: 370 mg | Sodium: 540 mg | Potassium: 700 mg

Cottage Cheese and Fruit Bowl

Serving: 4 | Prep time: 10 minutes | Cook time: 0 minutes

Ingredients:

- 16 oz (454 g) low-fat cottage cheese
- 8 oz (227 g) fresh mixed berries (strawberries, blueberries, raspberries)
- 4 oz (113 g) fresh pineapple chunks
- 4 oz (113 g) fresh mango chunks
- 2 oz (57 g) unsalted mixed nuts (almonds, walnuts, and cashews)
- 2 oz (57 g) honey
- 1 tsp vanilla extract
- 1/2 tsp ground cinnamon

Directions:

1. In a mixing bowl, combine the low-fat cottage cheese, honey, vanilla extract, and ground cinnamon. Mix until well combined.
2. Divide the sweetened cottage cheese mixture among four serving bowls.
3. Top each bowl with a generous portion of fresh mixed berries, fresh pineapple chunks, and fresh mango chunks.
4. Sprinkle a handful of unsalted mixed nuts over the fruit and cottage cheese.

Useful Tip: Customize your cottage cheese and fruit bowl with your favorite nuts or seeds for added crunch and texture, such as chia seeds or flaxseeds.

Nutritional Values: Calories: 280 kcal | Fat: 8 g | Protein: 18 g | Carbs: 38 g | Net carbs: 30 g | Fiber: 8 g | Cholesterol: 10 mg | Sodium: 420 mg | Potassium: 480 mg

Quinoa Breakfast Bowl with Almonds and Honey

Serving: 4 | Prep time: 10 minutes | Cook time: 20 minutes

Ingredients:

- 8 oz (227 g) quinoa
- 16 oz (473 ml) unsweetened almond milk
- 4 oz (113 g) almonds, chopped
- 2 oz (57 g) honey
- 1 oz (28 g) dried cranberries
- 1 tsp ground cinnamon
- 1/2 tsp vanilla extract
- Pinch of salt

Directions:

1. Rinse the quinoa under cold running water to remove any bitterness.
2. In a medium saucepan, combine the quinoa, salt and almond milk. Bring it to a boil over medium-high heat.
3. Reduce the heat to low, cover, and let it simmer for 15-20 minutes, or until the quinoa is tender and the liquid is absorbed. Fluff with a fork.
4. Stir in the vanilla extract and ground cinnamon into the cooked quinoa.
5. Divide the quinoa evenly among four serving bowls.
6. Top each bowl with chopped almonds and dried cranberries.
7. Drizzle honey over the quinoa and nut mixture for added sweetness.

Useful Tip: For extra creaminess, you can add a dollop of Greek yogurt on top of the quinoa before garnishing with almonds and honey.

Nutritional Values: Calories: 330 kcal | Fat: 11 g | Protein: 9 g | Carbs: 50 g | Net carbs: 39 g | Fiber: 11 g | Cholesterol: 0 mg | Sodium: 180 mg | Potassium: 430 mg

Zucchini and Carrot Fritters

Serving: 4 | Prep time: 15 minutes | Cook time: 20 minutes

Ingredients:

- 8 oz (227 g) zucchini, grated
- 8 oz (227 g) carrots, grated
- 4 oz (113 g) almond flour
- 2 oz (57 g) grated Parmesan cheese
- 2 large eggs
- 2 oz (57 g) fresh chives, finely chopped
- 2 oz (57 g) olive oil
- 1 tsp garlic powder
- Salt and pepper to taste

Directions:

1. Place the grated zucchini and carrots in a clean kitchen towel or cheesecloth, then squeeze to remove excess moisture.
2. In a mixing bowl, combine the grated zucchini and carrots, almond flour, grated Parmesan cheese, eggs, chopped chives, garlic powder, salt, and pepper. Mix until all ingredients are well combined.
3. Heat the olive oil in a large skillet over medium heat.
4. Scoop a spoonful of the fritter mixture and gently shape it into a patty using your hands. Place it in the hot skillet.
5. Repeat the process, adding as many patties as will comfortably fit in the skillet without overcrowding.
6. Cook the fritters for 3-4 minutes on each side, or until they are golden brown and crispy.
7. Transfer the cooked fritters to a paper towel-lined plate to remove any excess oil.

Useful Tip: To keep the fritters warm while cooking the entire batch, place them on a baking sheet in a preheated oven at 200°F (93°C).

Nutritional Values: Calories: 260 kcal | Fat: 19 g | Protein: 9 g | Carbs: 15 g | Net carbs: 9 g | Fiber: 6 g | Cholesterol: 95 mg | Sodium: 350 mg | Potassium: 440 mg

Veggie Ham and Cheese Omelette

Serving: 4 | Prep time: 10 minutes | Cook time: 10 minutes

Ingredients:

- 8 large eggs
- 4 oz (113 g) bell peppers, diced
- 1.2 oz (35 g) of ham, diced
- 4 oz (113 g) mushrooms, sliced
- 2 oz (57 g) red onion, finely chopped
- 2 oz (57 g) spinach leaves
- 4 oz (113 g) shredded low-fat cheddar cheese
- 2 oz (57 g) olive oil
- 1 tsp garlic powder
- Salt and pepper to taste

Directions:

1. In a large bowl, whisk together the eggs, garlic powder, salt, and pepper until well combined.
2. Heat 1 oz (28 g) of olive oil in a non-stick skillet over medium-high heat.
3. Add the diced bell peppers and chopped red onion to the skillet. Sauté for about 2-3 minutes until they begin to soften.
4. Stir in the sliced mushrooms and cook for an additional 2-3 minutes until they become tender.
5. Add the spinach leaves to the skillet and cook for 1-2 minutes until they wilt.
6. Transfer the cooked veggies to a plate and set them aside.
7. In the same skillet, add the remaining 1 oz (28 g) of olive oil and swirl it around to coat the bottom evenly.
8. Pour the whisked eggs and ham into the skillet, swirling to ensure an even distribution.
9. As the edges of the omelette start to set, use a spatula to gently lift the edges and tilt the skillet to allow the uncooked eggs to flow to the edges.
10. Once the eggs are mostly set but still slightly runny on top, sprinkle the shredded low-fat cheddar cheese over one-half of the omelette.
11. Carefully fold the other half of the omelette over the cheesy side.
12. Cook for an additional minute or until the cheese is melted and the omelette is cooked to your desired level of doneness.
13. Slide the omelette onto a serving plate and garnish with the sautéed vegetables.

Useful Tip: For a burst of freshness and flavor, top the omelette with a dollop of salsa or a sprinkle of fresh herbs such as cilantro or parsley before serving.

Nutritional Values: Calories: 250 kcal | Fat: 16 g | Protein: 18 g | Carbs: 8 g | Net carbs: 4 g | Fiber: 4 g | Cholesterol: 385 mg | Sodium: 290 mg | Potassium: 380 mg

Baked Apples with Cinnamon and Almonds

Serving: 4 | Prep time: 15 minutes | Cook time: 30 minutes

Ingredients:

- 4 medium-sized apples
- 4 oz (113 g) almonds, chopped
- 2 oz (57 g) honey
- 1 oz (28 g) unsalted butter, melted
- 1 tsp ground cinnamon
- 1/2 tsp vanilla extract
- 2 oz (57 g) water

Directions:

1. Preheat your oven to 350°F (175°C).

2. Wash the apples and use an apple corer to remove the cores while keeping the apples whole.

3. In a mixing bowl, combine the chopped almonds, honey, melted unsalted butter, ground cinnamon, and vanilla extract. Mix until you have a sticky almond mixture.

4. Stuff each apple with the almond mixture, packing it tightly into the cavity.

5. Place the stuffed apples in a baking dish.

6. Pour the water into the bottom of the baking dish to create steam while baking.

7. Cover the dish with aluminum foil and bake for 20 minutes.

8. Remove the foil and bake for an additional 10 minutes, or until the apples are tender and the almond stuffing is lightly browned.

Useful Tip: Serve the baked apples with a dollop of Greek yogurt or a scoop of low-fat vanilla ice cream for added creaminess and flavor.

Nutritional Values: Calories: 280 kcal | Fat: 15 g | Protein: 5 g | Carbs: 35 g | Net carbs: 28 g | Fiber: 7 g | Cholesterol: 10 mg | Sodium: 20 mg | Potassium: 380 mg

Turkey and Veggie Breakfast Casserole

Serving: 4 | Prep time: 15 minutes | Cook time: 30 minutes

Ingredients:

- 8 oz (227 g) ground turkey
- 4 oz (113 g) spinach leaves
- 4 oz (113 g) bell peppers, diced
- 2 oz (57 g) red onion, finely chopped
- 4 large eggs
- 4 oz (113 g) low-fat feta cheese, crumbled
- 4 oz (113 g) unsweetened almond milk
- 2 oz (57 g) olive oil
- 1 tsp garlic powder
- Salt and pepper to taste

Directions:

1. Preheat your oven to 350°F (175°C).

2. In a skillet, heat 1 oz (28 g) of olive oil over medium-high heat.

3. Add the ground turkey and cook, breaking it apart with a spatula, until it's browned and cooked through.

4. Remove the cooked turkey from the skillet and set it aside.

5. In the same skillet, add the remaining 1 oz (28 g) of olive oil and sauté the diced bell peppers and chopped red onion until they become tender, about 3-4 minutes.

6. Add the spinach leaves to the skillet and cook for an additional 1-2 minutes until they wilt.

7. In a mixing bowl, whisk together the eggs, almond milk, garlic powder, salt, and pepper.

8. In a greased baking dish, spread the cooked turkey evenly.

9. Layer the sautéed vegetables on top of the turkey.

10. Pour the egg mixture over the turkey and vegetables.

11. Sprinkle the crumbled low-fat feta cheese evenly over the top.

12. Bake in the preheated oven for 25-30 minutes or until the center is set and the edges are golden brown.

Useful Tip: Customize this casserole with your favorite veggies or herbs for added flavor and nutrition, such as diced tomatoes or fresh basil.

Nutritional Values: Calories: 320 kcal | Fat: 21 g | Protein: 22 g | Carbs: 11 g | Net carbs: 7 g | Fiber: 4 g | Cholesterol: 240 mg | Sodium: 450 mg | Potassium: 500 mg

Smoked Salmon and Cucumber Breakfast Wrap

Serving: 4 | Prep time: 10 minutes | Cook time: 5 minutes

Ingredients:

- 8 oz (227 g) smoked salmon slices
- 4 oz (113 g) cream cheese

- 4 large whole-wheat tortillas
- 4 oz (113 g) cucumber, thinly sliced
- 2 oz (57 g) red onion, thinly sliced
- 1 oz (28 g) fresh dill, chopped
- 1 tsp lemon zest
- Salt and pepper to taste

Directions:

1. In a small mixing bowl, combine the cream cheese, chopped fresh dill, lemon zest, salt, and pepper. Mix until well blended.
2. Lay out the whole-wheat tortillas on a clean surface.
3. Spread an even layer of the cream cheese mixture over each tortilla, leaving a small border around the edges.
4. Place a layer of smoked salmon slices on top of the cream cheese mixture.
5. Add a layer of thinly sliced cucumber and red onion on top of the salmon.
6. Carefully roll up each tortilla, tucking in the sides as you go to create a wrap.
7. Slice the wraps in half diagonally to make them easier to handle.

Useful Tip: For added flavor and a bit of heat, consider adding a touch of horseradish or a few capers to the cream cheese mixture.

Nutritional Values: Calories: 240 kcal | Fat: 10 g | Protein: 12 g | Carbs: 22 g | Net carbs: 18 g | Fiber: 4 g | Cholesterol: 30 mg | Sodium: 800 mg | Potassium: 330 mg

Spinach and Sun-Dried Tomato Quiche Cups

Serving: 4 | Prep time: 15 minutes | Cook time: 25 minutes

Ingredients:

- 4 large eggs
- 4 oz (113 g) fresh spinach, chopped
- 2 oz (57 g) sun-dried tomatoes, finely chopped
- 2 oz (57 g) feta cheese, crumbled
- 2 oz (57 g) milk
- 1 oz (28 g) olive oil
- 1 tsp dried oregano
- Salt and pepper to taste

Directions:

1. Preheat your oven to 350°F (175°C) and grease a muffin tin.
2. In a skillet, heat the olive oil over medium heat.
3. Add the chopped fresh spinach and sauté until wilted, about 2-3 minutes.
4. In a mixing bowl, whisk together the eggs, milk, dried oregano, salt, and pepper.
5. Stir in the finely chopped sun-dried tomatoes, crumbled feta cheese, and sautéed spinach.
6. Pour the egg mixture evenly into the greased muffin tin, filling each cup about 3/4 full.
7. Bake in the preheated oven for 20-25 minutes, or until the quiche cups are set and lightly browned on top.

Useful Tip: These quiche cups are versatile and can be made with other vegetables or cheeses according to your preference.

Nutritional Values: Calories: 190 kcal | Fat: 13 g | Protein: 9 g | Carbs: 7 g | Net carbs: 5 g | Fiber: 2 g | Cholesterol: 180 mg | Sodium: 350 mg | Potassium: 500 mg

SALADS

Grilled Chicken and Mixed Greens Salad

Serving: 4 | Prep time: 15 minutes | Cook time: 15 minutes

Ingredients:

- 16 oz (454 g) boneless, skinless chicken breasts
- 8 oz (227 g) mixed greens (e.g., spinach, arugula, and kale)
- 4 oz (113 g) cherry tomatoes, halved
- 2 oz (57 g) cucumber, sliced
- 2 oz (57 g) red onion, thinly sliced
- 1 oz (28 g) feta cheese, crumbled
- 1 oz (28 g) balsamic vinaigrette dressing
- 1 oz (28 g) olive oil
- 1 tsp dried oregano
- Salt and pepper to taste

Directions:

1. Preheat your grill to medium-high heat (around 400°F or 204°C).
2. Season the chicken breasts with olive oil, dried oregano, salt, and pepper.
3. Grill the chicken breasts for about 6-8 minutes per side, or until they reach an internal temperature of 165°F (74°C) and have grill marks. Remove from the grill and let them rest for a few minutes before slicing.
4. In a large salad bowl, combine the mixed greens, cherry tomatoes, sliced cucumber, and thinly sliced red onion.
5. Drizzle the balsamic vinaigrette dressing over the salad and toss to coat the ingredients evenly.
6. Divide the dressed salad among four plates.
7. Top each salad with sliced grilled chicken and crumbled feta cheese.

Useful Tip: To save time, you can use a store-bought balsamic vinaigrette dressing, or make your own by combining balsamic vinegar, olive oil, Dijon mustard, and honey.

Nutritional Values: Calories: 280 kcal | Fat: 16 g | Protein: 27 g | Carbs: 8 g | Net carbs: 5 g | Fiber: 3 g | Cholesterol: 75 mg | Sodium: 380 mg | Potassium: 600 mg

Quinoa and Roasted Vegetable Salad

Serving: 4 | Prep time: 15 minutes | Cook time: 25 minutes

Ingredients:

- 8 oz (227 g) quinoa
- 8 oz (227 g) bell peppers (assorted colors), diced
- 6 oz (170 g) zucchini, diced
- 6 oz (170 g) cherry tomatoes, halved
- 4 oz (113 g) red onion, diced
- 2 oz (57 g) black olives, sliced
- 2 oz (57 g) feta cheese, crumbled
- 2 oz (57 g) olive oil
- 1 oz (28 g) balsamic vinegar
- 1 tsp dried oregano
- Salt and pepper to taste
- Fresh basil leaves for garnish (optional)

Directions:

1. Preheat your oven to 400°F (204°C).
2. In a large bowl, toss the diced bell peppers, zucchini, cherry tomatoes, and red onion with olive oil, dried oregano, salt, and pepper.
3. Spread the seasoned vegetables evenly on a baking sheet and roast in the preheated oven for about 20-25 minutes or until they are tender and slightly caramelized. Stir them once or twice during roasting.
4. While the vegetables are roasting, rinse the quinoa under cold water. In a medium saucepan, combine the quinoa with 16 oz (473 ml) of water. Bring to a boil, then reduce the heat, cover, and simmer for about 15 minutes, or until the water is absorbed. Fluff the cooked quinoa with a fork and let it cool.
5. In a large salad bowl, combine the cooked quinoa, roasted vegetables, sliced black olives, and crumbled

feta cheese.

6. Drizzle balsamic vinegar over the salad and toss to combine all the ingredients.

7. Garnish with fresh basil leaves if desired.

Useful Tip: You can customize this salad with your favorite roasted vegetables, such as eggplant, asparagus, or carrots.

Nutritional Values: Calories: 375 kcal | Fat: 18 g | Protein: 10 g | Carbs: 43 g | Net carbs: 33 g | Fiber: 10 g | Cholesterol: 13 mg | Sodium: 421 mg | Potassium: 593 mg

Tuna and White Bean Salad

Serving: 4 | Prep time: 15 minutes | Cook time: 0 minutes

Ingredients:

- 12 oz (340 g) canned tuna, drained
- 12 oz (340 g) canned white beans, drained and rinsed
- 4 oz (113 g) red onion, finely chopped
- 4 oz (113 g) celery, finely chopped
- 2 oz (57 g) fresh parsley, chopped
- 2 oz (57 g) olive oil
- 2 oz (57 g) lemon juice
- 1 oz (28 g) Dijon mustard
- Salt and pepper to taste

Directions:

1. In a large bowl, combine the drained tuna, white beans, finely chopped red onion, celery, and fresh parsley.

2. In a separate small bowl, whisk together the olive oil, lemon juice, and Dijon mustard until well combined.

3. Pour the dressing over the tuna and white bean mixture and gently toss to coat all the ingredients.

4. Season the salad with salt and pepper to taste. Adjust the seasoning as needed.

5. Allow the salad to marinate in the refrigerator for at least 30 minutes before serving to let the flavors meld together.

Useful Tip: This salad is even better the next day, so consider making it in advance for a quick and healthy meal.

Nutritional Values: Calories: 320 kcal | Fat: 14 g | Protein: 31 g | Carbs: 20 g | Net carbs: 14 g | Fiber: 6 g | Cholesterol: 42 mg | Sodium: 610 mg | Potassium: 690 mg

Spinach and Strawberry Salad

Serving: 4 | Prep time: 15 minutes | Cook time: 0 minutes

Ingredients:

- 8 oz (227 g) fresh baby spinach leaves
- 8 oz (227 g) fresh strawberries, hulled and sliced
- 2 oz (57 g) red onion, thinly sliced
- 2 oz (57 g) feta cheese, crumbled
- 2 oz (57 g) toasted pecans, chopped
- 2 oz (57 g) balsamic vinaigrette dressing
- 1 oz (28 g) extra-virgin olive oil
- 1 oz (28 g) balsamic glaze (for drizzling)
- Salt and pepper to taste

Directions:

1. In a large salad bowl, combine the fresh baby spinach leaves, sliced strawberries, thinly sliced red onion, crumbled feta cheese, and chopped toasted pecans.

2. In a separate small bowl, whisk together the balsamic vinaigrette dressing and extra-virgin olive oil until well blended.

3. Drizzle the dressing over the salad mixture, ensuring even distribution.

4. Season the salad with salt and pepper to taste. Adjust the seasoning as needed.

5. Lightly toss the salad to coat the ingredients with the dressing, being careful not to crush the delicate spinach leaves.

6. Drizzle balsamic glaze over the top of the salad for added sweetness and presentation.

Useful Tip: For added protein, consider adding grilled chicken or shrimp to make this salad a complete meal.

Nutritional Values: Calories: 220 kcal | Fat: 17 g | Protein: 4 g | Carbs: 15 g | Net carbs: 10 g | Fiber: 5 g | Cholesterol: 8 mg | Sodium: 310 mg | Potassium: 430 mg

Cucumber and Tomato Salad with Dill Yogurt Dressing

Serving: 4 | Prep time: 15 minutes | Cook time: 0 minutes

Ingredients:

- 8 oz (227 g) cucumber, thinly sliced
- 8 oz (227 g) cherry tomatoes, halved
- 2 oz (57 g) red onion, thinly sliced
- 2 oz (57 g) Greek yogurt
- 1 oz (28 g) fresh dill, chopped

- 1 oz (28 g) lemon juice
- 1 oz (28 g) extra-virgin olive oil
- 1 oz (28 g) honey
- Salt and pepper to taste

Directions:

1. In a large salad bowl, combine the thinly sliced cucumber, halved cherry tomatoes, and thinly sliced red onion.
2. In a separate bowl, whisk together the Greek yogurt, fresh dill, lemon juice, extra-virgin olive oil, honey, salt, and pepper until the dressing is well blended.
3. Pour the dill yogurt dressing over the cucumber, tomato, and onion mixture.
4. Gently toss the salad to ensure even distribution of the dressing without crushing the ingredients.

Useful Tip: To enhance the flavor, consider adding crumbled feta cheese or chopped Kalamata olives as optional toppings.

Nutritional Values: Calories: 100 kcal | Fat: 6 g | Protein: 2 g | Carbs: 10 g | Net carbs: 7 g | Fiber: 3 g | Cholesterol: 0 mg | Sodium: 60 mg | Potassium: 290 mg

Mango and Avocado Salad

Serving: 4 | Prep time: 15 minutes | Cook time: 0 minutes

Ingredients:

- 8 oz (227 g) mango, peeled, pitted, and diced
- 8 oz (227 g) avocado, peeled, pitted, and diced
- 2 oz (57 g) red onion, finely chopped
- 2 oz (57 g) fresh cilantro, chopped

- 1 oz (28 g) lime juice
- 1 oz (28 g) extra-virgin olive oil
- 1 oz (28 g) honey
- Salt and pepper to taste

Directions:

1. In a large salad bowl, combine the diced mango, diced avocado, finely chopped red onion, and fresh cilantro.
2. In a separate bowl, whisk together the lime juice, extra-virgin olive oil, honey, salt, and pepper to create the dressing.
3. Pour the dressing over the mango, avocado, onion, and cilantro mixture.
4. Gently toss the salad to ensure the dressing evenly coats all the ingredients.

Useful Tip: For a touch of heat, consider adding a pinch of crushed red pepper flakes or finely diced jalapeño pepper to the salad.

Nutritional Values: Calories: 180 kcal | Fat: 12 g | Protein: 2 g | Carbs: 21 g | Net carbs: 15 g | Fiber: 6 g | Cholesterol: 0 mg | Sodium: 120 mg | Potassium: 470 mg

Chickpea and Cucumber Salad

Serving: 4 | Prep time: 15 minutes | Cook time: 0 minutes

Ingredients:

- 8 oz (227 g) canned chickpeas, drained and rinsed
- 8 oz (227 g) cucumber, diced
- 2 oz (57 g) red bell pepper, finely chopped
- 2 oz (57 g) red onion, finely chopped
- 2 oz (57 g) fresh parsley, chopped
- 1 oz (28 g) lemon juice
- 1 oz (28 g) extra-virgin olive oil
- 1 oz (28 g) red wine vinegar
- Salt and pepper to taste

Directions:

1. In a large salad bowl, combine the drained and rinsed chickpeas, diced cucumber, finely chopped red bell pepper, finely chopped red onion, and fresh parsley.
2. In a separate bowl, whisk together the lemon juice, extra-virgin olive oil, red wine vinegar, salt, and pepper to create the dressing.
3. Pour the dressing over the chickpea and vegetable mixture.
4. Gently toss the salad to ensure the dressing evenly coats all the ingredients.

Useful Tip: To add an extra layer of flavor, consider adding crumbled feta cheese or Kalamata olives to the salad.

Nutritional Values: Calories: 190 kcal | Fat: 10 g | Protein: 5 g | Carbs: 20 g | Net carbs: 13 g | Fiber: 7 g | Cholesterol: 0 mg | Sodium: 280 mg | Potassium: 290 mg

Kale and Pomegranate Salad

Serving: 4 | Prep time: 15 minutes | Cook time: 0 minutes

Ingredients:

- 8 oz (227 g) fresh kale, stems removed and leaves torn into bite-sized pieces
- 4 oz (113 g) pomegranate seeds
- 2 oz (57 g) toasted walnuts, roughly chopped
- 2 oz (57 g) crumbled goat cheese
- 1 oz (28 g) extra-virgin olive oil
- 1 oz (28 g) lemon juice
- 1 oz (28 g) honey
- Salt and pepper to taste

Directions:

1. In a large salad bowl, place the torn kale leaves.
2. In a separate small bowl, whisk together the lemon juice, honey, extra-virgin olive oil, salt, and pepper to create the dressing.
3. Pour the dressing over the kale leaves and massage it into the leaves with clean hands for a few minutes until the kale begins to soften.
4. Add the pomegranate seeds, toasted walnuts, and crumbled goat cheese to the salad.

Useful Tip: For a slightly sweeter variation, you can substitute maple syrup for honey in the dressing.

Nutritional Values: Calories: 250 kcal | Fat: 15 g | Protein: 7 g | Carbs: 24 g | Net carbs: 17 g | Fiber: 7 g | Cholesterol: 10 mg | Sodium: 120 mg | Potassium: 560 mg

Roasted Beet and Goat Cheese Salad

Serving: 4 | Prep time: 15 minutes | Cook time: 45 minutes

Ingredients:

- 16 oz (454 g) beets, peeled and cut into bite-sized pieces
- 2 oz (57 g) olive oil
- Salt and pepper to taste
- 4 oz (113 g) mixed greens (such as arugula, spinach, and kale)

- 4 oz (113 g) goat cheese, crumbled
- 2 oz (57 g) balsamic vinegar
- 1 oz (28 g) honey
- 2 oz (57 g) chopped walnuts, toasted

Directions:

1. Preheat the oven to 400°F (200°C).
2. Toss the beet pieces with olive oil, salt, and pepper on a baking sheet. Roast in the preheated oven for about 45 minutes or until the beets are tender and slightly caramelized.
3. While the beets are roasting, prepare the dressing by whisking together the balsamic vinegar, honey, and a pinch of salt and pepper in a small bowl.
4. Once the beets are done roasting, let them cool slightly.
5. In a large salad bowl, place the mixed greens.
6. Add the roasted beets, crumbled goat cheese, and toasted walnuts to the greens.
7. Drizzle the balsamic dressing over the salad and toss gently to combine.

Useful Tip: You can save time by using pre-cooked beets available in many grocery stores.

Nutritional Values: Calories: 320 kcal | Fat: 22 g | Protein: 8 g | Carbs: 26 g | Net carbs: 22 g | Fiber: 4 g | Cholesterol: 20 mg | Sodium: 240 mg | Potassium: 680 mg

Broccoli and Cranberry Salad

Serving: 4 | Prep time: 15 minutes | Cook time: 0 minutes

Ingredients:

- 12 oz (340 g) broccoli florets, blanched and chopped
- 2 oz (57 g) dried cranberries
- 2 oz (57 g) red onion, finely chopped
- 2 oz (57 g) sunflower seeds
- 2 oz (57 g) Greek yogurt

- 2 oz (57 g) mayonnaise
- 2 oz (57 g) apple cider vinegar
- 1 oz (28 g) honey
- Salt and pepper to taste

Directions:

1. In a large mixing bowl, combine the blanched and chopped broccoli florets, dried cranberries, chopped red onion, and sunflower seeds.
2. In a separate bowl, whisk together the Greek yogurt, mayonnaise, apple cider vinegar, honey, salt, and pepper to create the dressing.
3. Pour the dressing over the broccoli mixture and toss to coat all the ingredients evenly.
4. Refrigerate the salad for at least 30 minutes to allow the flavors to meld together.

Useful Tip: You can blanch the broccoli by briefly immersing it in boiling water for about 2 minutes and then immediately cooling it in ice water to maintain its vibrant green color and crisp texture.

Nutritional Values: Calories: 230 kcal | Fat: 14 g | Protein: 4 g | Carbs: 24 g | Net carbs: 19 g | Fiber: 5 g | Cholesterol: 10 mg | Sodium: 180 mg | Potassium: 360 mg

Pear and Walnut Salad

Serving: 4 | Prep time: 10 minutes | Cook time: 0 minutes

Ingredients:

- 12 oz (340 g) mixed salad greens
- 2 ripe pears, thinly sliced
- 2 oz (57 g) chopped walnuts
- 2 oz (57 g) crumbled blue cheese
- 2 oz (57 g) balsamic vinaigrette dressing
- 1 oz (28 ml) extra-virgin olive oil
- Salt and pepper to taste

Directions:

1. In a large salad bowl, combine the mixed salad greens, thinly sliced pears, chopped walnuts, and crumbled blue cheese.
2. In a separate bowl, whisk together the balsamic vinaigrette dressing, extra-virgin olive oil, salt, and pepper to create the salad dressing.
3. Drizzle the dressing over the salad ingredients.
4. Toss everything together gently to ensure the salad is evenly coated with the dressing.

Useful Tip: To prevent the pears from browning, you can toss them in a bit of lemon juice before adding them to the salad.

Nutritional Values: Calories: 250 kcal | Fat: 18 g | Protein: 5 g | Carbs: 20 g | Net carbs: 15 g | Fiber: 5 g | Cholesterol: 10 mg | Sodium: 350 mg | Potassium: 380 mg

Asian-Inspired Chicken Salad

Serving: 4 | Prep time: 15 minutes | Cook time: 15 minutes

Ingredients:

- 16 oz (450 g) boneless, skinless chicken breasts
- 8 oz (227 g) mixed salad greens
- 2 oz (57 g) sliced almonds
- 2 oz (57 g) shredded carrots
- 2 oz (57 g) sliced cucumber
- 2 oz (57 g) edamame (cooked and shelled)
- 2 oz (57 g) red bell pepper, thinly sliced
- 2 oz (57 g) green onions, chopped
- Salt and pepper to taste

For the Dressing:

- 2 oz (57 ml) low-sodium soy sauce
- 1 oz (28 ml) rice vinegar
- 1 oz (28 ml) sesame oil
- 1 oz (28 ml) honey
- 1 tsp fresh ginger, minced
- 1 tsp fresh garlic, minced
- Sesame seeds for garnish (optional)

Directions:

1. Preheat a grill or grill pan to medium-high heat. Season the chicken breasts with salt and pepper. Grill for about 6-7 minutes per side or until the chicken is cooked through. Remove from heat, let it rest for a few minutes, and then slice it into thin strips.
2. In a large salad bowl, combine the mixed salad greens, sliced almonds, shredded carrots, sliced cucumber, edamame, red bell pepper, and chopped green onions.
3. In a separate bowl, whisk together the low-sodium soy sauce, rice vinegar, sesame oil, honey, minced ginger, and minced garlic to create the dressing.
4. Drizzle the dressing over the salad ingredients and toss everything together until well combined.
5. Top the salad with the grilled chicken slices and garnish with sesame seeds if desired.

Useful Tip: To make this salad even more refreshing, you can chill it in the refrigerator for about 30 minutes before serving.

Nutritional Values: Calories: 350 kcal | Fat: 15 g | Protein: 28 g | Carbs: 26 g | Net carbs: 18 g | Fiber: 8 g | Cholesterol: 65 mg | Sodium: 700 mg | Potassium: 780 mg

Roasted Butternut Squash and Quinoa Salad

Serving: 4 | Prep time: 15 minutes | Cook time: 25 minutes

Ingredients:

- 16 oz (450 g) butternut squash, peeled, seeded, and cubed
- 8 oz (227 g) quinoa
- 2 oz (57 g) baby spinach
- 2 oz (57 g) dried cranberries
- 2 oz (57 g) pumpkin seeds
- 2 oz (57 g) crumbled feta cheese
- 2 oz (57 ml) olive oil
- 1 oz (28 ml) balsamic vinegar
- 1 tsp honey
- Salt and pepper to taste
- 1/2 tsp dried thyme (optional)
- Fresh parsley for garnish (optional)

Directions:

1. Preheat your oven to 400°F (200°C).
2. In a bowl, toss the cubed butternut squash with 1 tablespoon of olive oil, salt, pepper, and dried thyme if desired. Spread the squash on a baking sheet and roast in the preheated oven for about 20-25 minutes or until it's tender and slightly caramelized. Remove from the oven and let it cool.
3. While the butternut squash is roasting, rinse the quinoa under cold water, and cook it according to the package instructions. Once cooked, fluff it with a fork and allow it to cool.
4. In a small bowl, whisk together the remaining olive oil, balsamic vinegar, honey, salt, and pepper to create the dressing.
5. In a large salad bowl, combine the cooked quinoa, roasted butternut squash, baby spinach, dried cranberries, and pumpkin seeds.
6. Drizzle the dressing over the salad and gently toss to coat all the ingredients.
7. Top the salad with crumbled feta cheese and garnish with fresh parsley if desired.

Useful Tip: This salad can be served warm or at room temperature, making it a versatile and satisfying dish.

Nutritional Values: Calories: 380 kcal | Fat: 17 g | Protein: 10 g | Carbs: 51 g | Net carbs: 43 g | Fiber: 8 g | Cholesterol: 10 mg | Sodium: 160 mg | Potassium: 670 mg

Egg Salad with Greens

Serving: 4 | Prep time: 10 minutes | Cook time: 10 minutes

Ingredients:

- 8 large eggs
- 4 oz (113 g) mixed greens (e.g., spinach, arugula, and kale)
- 1 oz (28 g) cherry tomatoes, halved
- 1 oz (28 g) cucumber, sliced
- 1 oz (28 g) red bell pepper, diced
- 1 oz (28 g) red onion, finely chopped
- 2 oz (57 ml) Greek yogurt
- 1 oz (28 ml) olive oil
- 1 oz (28 ml) lemon juice
- 1 tsp Dijon mustard
- Salt and pepper to taste
- 1/2 tsp dried dill (optional)
- Fresh chives for garnish (optional)

Directions:

1. Place the eggs in a saucepan and cover them with water. Bring the water to a boil, then reduce the heat to a simmer and cook for 9-12 minutes, depending on your desired yolk consistency (9 minutes for soft-boiled, 12 minutes for hard-boiled).
2. While the eggs are cooking, prepare an ice bath by filling a large bowl with ice and cold water. When the eggs are done, immediately transfer them to the ice bath to cool for a few minutes. This helps in easy peeling.

3. Once the eggs are cooled, peel and chop them into bite-sized pieces.

4. In a large salad bowl, combine the mixed greens, cherry tomatoes, cucumber, red bell pepper, and red onion.

5. In a separate bowl, whisk together the Greek yogurt, olive oil, lemon juice, Dijon mustard, salt, and pepper to create the dressing. Add dried dill for extra flavor if desired.

6. Add the chopped eggs to the salad bowl and drizzle the dressing over the salad. Toss gently to coat all the ingredients with the dressing.

7. Garnish with fresh chives if desired.

Useful Tip: To make peeling the eggs even easier, you can add a teaspoon of vinegar to the boiling water.

Nutritional Values: Calories: 240 kcal | Fat: 18 g | Protein: 13 g | Carbs: 7 g | Net carbs: 5 g | Fiber: 2 g | Cholesterol: 380 mg | Sodium: 250 mg | Potassium: 320 mg

Black Bean and Corn Salad

Serving: 4 | Prep time: 15 minutes | Cook time: 0 minutes

Ingredients:

- 14 oz (400 g) can of black beans, drained and rinsed
- 8 oz (227 g) canned corn, drained (or use fresh corn kernels if available)
- 1 red bell pepper, diced
- 1/2 red onion, finely chopped
- 1 jalapeño pepper, seeds removed and finely chopped (adjust to your preferred spice level)
- 2 oz (57 ml) fresh lime juice
- 2 oz (57 ml) olive oil
- 1 tsp ground cumin
- Salt and pepper to taste
- 2 oz (57 ml) fresh cilantro, chopped (optional)
- Avocado slices for garnish (optional)

Directions:

1. In a large mixing bowl, combine the black beans, corn, diced red bell pepper, finely chopped red onion, and jalapeño pepper.

2. In a separate bowl, whisk together the fresh lime juice, olive oil, ground cumin, salt, and pepper to create the dressing.

3. Pour the dressing over the bean and vegetable mixture. Toss everything together gently to coat the ingredients evenly with the dressing.

4. If you like cilantro, sprinkle it over the salad and gently mix.

5. If desired, garnish the salad with slices of ripe avocado.

Useful Tip: For extra flavor, let the salad sit in the refrigerator for at least 30 minutes before serving to allow the flavors to meld.

Nutritional Values: Calories: 320 kcal | Fat: 16 g | Protein: 9 g | Carbs: 39 g | Net carbs: 30 g | Fiber: 9 g | Cholesterol: 0 mg | Sodium: 480 mg | Potassium: 660 mg

Mediterranean Cucumber and Feta Salad

Serving: 4 | Prep time: 15 minutes | Cook time: 0 minutes

Ingredients:

- 14 oz (400 g) cucumber, thinly sliced
- 7 oz (200 g) cherry tomatoes, halved
- 4 oz (115 g) feta cheese, crumbled
- 1/4 red onion, thinly sliced
- 2 tbsp extra virgin olive oil
- 1 oz (30 ml) lemon juice
- 1/2 tsp dried oregano
- Salt and pepper to taste
- Fresh parsley for garnish, chopped
- Kalamata olives for garnish (optional)

Directions:

1. In a large bowl, combine the thinly sliced cucumber, halved cherry tomatoes, crumbled feta cheese, and thinly sliced red onion.

2. In a small bowl, whisk together the extra virgin olive oil, lemon juice, dried oregano, salt, and pepper to make the dressing.

3. Pour the dressing over the cucumber mixture and toss gently to coat everything evenly.

4. Garnish the salad with chopped fresh parsley and, if desired, Kalamata olives.

Useful Tip: To enhance the flavors, let the salad marinate in the refrigerator for about 30 minutes before serving.

Nutritional Values: Calories: 180 kcal | Fat: 14 g | Protein: 6 g | Carbs: 8 g | Net carbs: 5 g | Fiber: 3 g | Cholesterol: 25 mg | Sodium: 330 mg | Potassium: 320 mg

SNACKS

Trail Mix with Nuts and Dried Fruit

Serving: 4 | Prep time: 10 minutes | Cook time: 0 minutes

Ingredients:

- 4 oz (113 g) almonds
- 4 oz (113 g) walnuts
- 2 oz (57 g) dried cranberries
- 2 oz (57 g) raisins
- 2 oz (57 g) dried apricots, chopped
- 2 oz (57 g) dark chocolate chips (70% cocoa or higher)
- 1/2 tsp ground cinnamon
- 1/4 tsp sea salt

Directions:

1. In a large bowl, combine the almonds, walnuts, dried cranberries, raisins, chopped dried apricots, and dark chocolate chips.
2. Sprinkle ground cinnamon and sea salt over the mixture.
3. Gently toss all the ingredients until well combined.
4. Transfer the trail mix to an airtight container or portion it into snack-sized bags for easy on-the-go enjoyment.

Useful Tip: Customize your trail mix by adding your favorite nuts, seeds, or dried fruits to suit your taste preferences.

Nutritional Values: Calories: 400 kcal | Fat: 28 g | Protein: 9 g | Carbs: 34 g | Net carbs: 22 g | Fiber: 12 g | Cholesterol: 0 mg | Sodium: 110 mg | Potassium: 440 mg

Carrot and Cucumber Sticks with Tzatziki Dip

Serving: 4 | Prep time: 15 minutes | Cook time: 0 minutes

Ingredients:

- 2 medium carrots, peeled and cut into sticks
- 2 medium cucumbers, cut into sticks
- 8 oz (226 g) Greek yogurt
- 1/2 cucumber, finely grated and drained
- 1 clove garlic, minced
- 1 tbsp lemon juice
- 1 tbsp olive oil
- 1 tsp fresh dill, chopped
- Salt and pepper to taste

Directions:

1. Prepare the carrot and cucumber sticks by cutting them into bite-sized pieces.
2. In a mixing bowl, combine Greek yogurt, finely grated and drained cucumber, minced garlic, lemon juice, olive oil, and fresh dill. Mix until well combined.
3. Season the tzatziki dip with salt and pepper to taste, adjusting the seasoning as needed.
4. Arrange the carrot and cucumber sticks on a serving platter.
5. Serve the tzatziki dip alongside the carrot and cucumber sticks for dipping.

Useful Tip: For a creamier tzatziki, refrigerate the dip for about an hour before serving to allow the flavors to meld.

Nutritional Values: Calories: 85 kcal | Fat: 4 g | Protein: 5 g | Carbs: 9 g | Net carbs: 5 g | Fiber: 4 g | Cholesterol: 3 mg | Sodium: 27 mg | Potassium: 333 mg

Cherry Tomatoes with Fresh Mozzarella

Serving: 4 | Prep time: 10 minutes | Cook time: 0 minutes

Ingredients:

- 8 oz (226 g) cherry tomatoes
- 8 oz (226 g) fresh mozzarella cheese balls
- 2 tbsp extra-virgin olive oil
- 1 tbsp balsamic vinegar
- Fresh basil leaves for garnish
- Salt and pepper to taste

Directions:

1. Rinse and dry the cherry tomatoes, and then cut them in half.
2. Drain the fresh mozzarella cheese balls and pat them dry with a paper towel.
3. In a large bowl, combine the cherry tomatoes and fresh mozzarella cheese balls.
4. In a small bowl, whisk together the extra-virgin olive oil and balsamic vinegar to create a simple vinaigrette.
5. Drizzle the vinaigrette over the cherry tomatoes and mozzarella. Gently toss to coat.
6. Season with salt and pepper to taste.
7. Garnish the dish with fresh basil leaves.

Useful Tip: For added flavor, marinate the cherry tomatoes and mozzarella in the vinaigrette for about 15 minutes before serving.

Nutritional Values: Calories: 240 kcal | Fat: 20 g | Protein: 12 g | Carbs: 4 g | Net carbs: 3 g | Fiber: 1 g | Cholesterol: 45 mg | Sodium: 400 mg | Potassium: 200 mg

Celery Stuffed with Cream Cheese and Raisins

Serving: 4 | Prep time: 15 minutes | Cook time: 0 minutes

Ingredients:

- 4 oz (113 g) cream cheese, softened
- 1 oz (28 g) raisins
- 8 celery stalks, washed and trimmed
- 1 tsp honey
- 1/2 tsp lemon juice
- Pinch of salt

Directions:

1. In a mixing bowl, combine the softened cream cheese, raisins, honey, lemon juice, and a pinch of salt. Mix until well blended.
2. Using a small spoon or a butter knife, carefully fill each celery stalk with the cream cheese mixture, spreading it evenly.
3. Place the stuffed celery stalks on a serving platter.
4. Garnish with additional raisins or a drizzle of honey, if desired.

Useful Tip: For a crunchier texture, you can refrigerate the stuffed celery for about 30 minutes before serving.

Nutritional Values: Calories: 160 kcal | Fat: 12 g | Protein: 2 g | Carbs: 11 g | Net carbs: 9 g | Fiber: 2 g | Cholesterol: 40 mg | Sodium: 160 mg | Potassium: 270 mg

Spinach and Feta Stuffed Mushrooms

Serving: 4 | Prep time: 20 minutes | Cook time: 20 minutes

Ingredients:

- 16 large button mushrooms, stems removed and reserved
- 4 oz (113 g) fresh spinach, chopped
- 2 oz (57 g) feta cheese, crumbled
- 2 cloves garlic, minced
- 1 tbsp olive oil
- Salt and pepper, to taste
- 1/2 tsp lemon juice
- 1/2 tsp dried oregano

- Cooking spray

Directions:

1. Preheat your oven to 375°F (190°C).

2. Clean the mushroom caps and set them aside. Chop the reserved mushroom stems finely.

3. In a skillet, heat the olive oil over medium heat. Add the minced garlic and chopped mushroom stems. Sauté until they release their moisture and become tender, about 5 minutes.

4. Add the chopped spinach to the skillet and cook until wilted, about 2-3 minutes. Season with salt, pepper, lemon juice, and dried oregano. Stir well.

5. Remove the skillet from heat and let it cool slightly. Once cooled, mix in the crumbled feta cheese.

6. Generously fill each mushroom cap with the spinach and feta mixture.

7. Place the stuffed mushrooms on a baking sheet coated with cooking spray.

8. Bake in the preheated oven for approximately 15-20 minutes or until the mushrooms are tender and the filling is golden on top.

Useful Tip: For a golden-brown crust on top, you can broil the stuffed mushrooms for the last 1-2 minutes of baking.

Nutritional Values: Calories: 80 kcal | Fat: 5 g | Protein: 4 g | Carbs: 5 g | Net carbs: 3 g | Fiber: 2 g | Cholesterol: 11 mg | Sodium: 180 mg | Potassium: 400 mg

Yogurt and Cucumber Dip with Pita Wedges

Serving: 4 | Prep time: 15 minutes | Cook time: 0 minutes

Ingredients:

- 8 oz (227 g) Greek yogurt
- 1 medium cucumber, finely grated
- 2 cloves garlic, minced
- 2 tbsp fresh lemon juice
- 1 tbsp extra-virgin olive oil
- 1 tsp dried dill
- Salt and pepper, to taste
- 4 whole wheat pita bread, cut into wedges

Directions:

1. In a mixing bowl, combine the Greek yogurt, grated cucumber, minced garlic, fresh lemon juice, and extra-virgin olive oil. Mix until well combined.

2. Add the dried dill, salt, and pepper to the yogurt mixture. Stir thoroughly, ensuring all ingredients are evenly incorporated.

3. Taste the dip and adjust the seasoning if needed, adding more salt, pepper, or lemon juice to your preference.

4. Cover the bowl and refrigerate the yogurt and cucumber dip for at least 30 minutes to allow the flavors to meld.

5. While the dip is chilling, preheat your oven to 350°F (175°C).

6. Place the pita wedges on a baking sheet and lightly toast them in the oven for about 5-7 minutes or until they become crisp.

7. Serve the chilled yogurt and cucumber dip alongside the toasted whole wheat pita wedges.

Useful Tip: For added flavor, you can sprinkle some additional dried dill or a drizzle of olive oil on top of the dip before serving.

Nutritional Values: Calories: 180 kcal | Fat: 4 g | Protein: 9 g | Carbs: 28 g | Net carbs: 24 g | Fiber: 4 g | Cholesterol: 3 mg | Sodium: 260 mg | Potassium: 245 mg

Edamame with Sea Salt

Serving: 4 | Prep time: 5 minutes | Cook time: 5 minutes

Ingredients:

- 16 oz (450 g) frozen edamame (in pods)
- 2 tsp sea salt

Directions:

1. In a large pot, bring water to a boil.
2. Add the frozen edamame pods to the boiling water.
3. Boil for about 5 minutes, or until the edamame pods are tender.
4. Drain the cooked edamame in a colander.
5. While the edamame are still hot, sprinkle them with sea salt.
6. Toss the edamame to ensure that the sea salt coats them evenly.
7. Serve the edamame with sea salt immediately as a healthy and satisfying snack.

Useful Tip: To enjoy the edamame, simply squeeze the pods to release the beans into your mouth. Discard the empty pods.

Nutritional Values: Calories: 130 kcal | Fat: 4 g | Protein: 11 g | Carbs: 14 g | Net carbs: 5 g | Fiber: 9 g | Cholesterol: 0 mg | Sodium: 470 mg | Potassium: 340 mg

Roasted Chickpeas

Serving: 4 | Prep time: 5 minutes | Cook time: 30 minutes

Ingredients:

- 15 oz (425 g) canned chickpeas, drained and rinsed
- 2 tbsp olive oil
- 1/2 tsp smoked paprika
- 1/2 tsp cumin
- 1/4 tsp cayenne pepper (adjust to taste)
- 1/2 tsp garlic powder
- Salt and pepper to taste

Directions:

1. Preheat your oven to 400°F (200°C).
2. In a mixing bowl, combine the drained and rinsed chickpeas, olive oil, smoked paprika, cumin, cayenne pepper, garlic powder, salt, and pepper. Toss until the chickpeas are well-coated with the seasoning.
3. Spread the seasoned chickpeas in a single layer on a baking sheet.
4. Roast in the preheated oven for about 30 minutes or until the chickpeas become crispy and golden brown. Shake the pan or stir the chickpeas every 10 minutes for even roasting.
5. Remove from the oven and let them cool slightly before serving.

Useful Tip: Roasted chickpeas are a great crunchy snack, but they can also be used as a topping for salads or a side dish for your favorite meal.

Nutritional Values: Calories: 180 kcal | Fat: 7 g | Protein: 6 g | Carbs: 21 g | Net carbs: 13 g | Fiber: 8 g | Cholesterol: 0 mg | Sodium: 240 mg | Potassium: 190 mg

Cucumber and Avocado Sushi Rolls

Serving: 4 | Prep time: 20 minutes | Cook time: 15 minutes

Ingredients:

- 7 oz (200 g) sushi rice
- 16 oz (480 ml) water
- 4 sheets nori (seaweed) sheets
- 1 avocado, thinly sliced
- 1 cucumber, thinly sliced
- 2 oz (60 ml) rice vinegar
- 1 tbsp sugar
- 1 tsp salt
- Soy sauce and wasabi for dipping (optional)
- Pickled ginger for serving (optional)

Directions:

1. Rinse the sushi rice in a fine-mesh strainer until the water runs clear.

2. In a medium saucepan, combine the sushi rice and 2 cups of water. Bring to a boil, then reduce the heat to low, cover, and simmer for 15 minutes, or until the rice is cooked and the water is absorbed.

3. While the rice is cooking, in a small bowl, mix the rice vinegar, sugar, and salt until dissolved. When the rice is done, transfer it to a large bowl and drizzle the vinegar mixture over it. Gently toss the rice to evenly coat it with the seasoned vinegar. Allow it to cool to room temperature.

4. Lay a bamboo sushi rolling mat on a clean surface, and place a sheet of plastic wrap on top of it.

5. Lay a nori sheet, shiny side down, on the plastic wrap-covered sushi rolling mat.

6. Wet your hands to prevent sticking, then take a handful of sushi rice and evenly spread it over the nori, leaving about 1/2 inch (1.25 cm) of nori on the far side.

7. Lay avocado and cucumber slices evenly over the rice.

8. Carefully lift the bamboo mat and start rolling the nori and rice over the avocado and cucumber, using gentle pressure to form a tight roll. Roll until you reach the exposed edge of the nori, then moisten the edge with a bit of water to seal the roll.

9. Using a sharp knife dipped in water, slice the roll into bite-sized pieces.

10. Repeat the process with the remaining nori sheets and ingredients.

11. Serve your cucumber and avocado sushi rolls with soy sauce, wasabi, and pickled ginger if desired.

Useful Tip: To prevent the rice from sticking to your hands while spreading it on the nori, keep a small bowl of water nearby to dip your fingers into.

Nutritional Values: Calories: 220 kcal | Fat: 7 g | Protein: 3 g | Carbs: 37 g | Net carbs: 30 g | Fiber: 7 g | Cholesterol: 0 mg | Sodium: 590 mg | Potassium: 450 mg

Carrot and Hummus Pinwheels

Serving: 4 | Prep time: 15 minutes | Cook time: 0 minutes

Ingredients:

- 4 large whole wheat tortillas
- 3.5 oz (100 g) shredded carrots
- 4.2 oz (120 g) hummus
- 1.1 oz (30 g) chopped fresh spinach
- 1.1 oz (30 g) diced red bell pepper
- 1.1 oz (30 g) diced cucumber
- 1.1 oz (30 g) diced red onion
- 0.2 oz (5 g) lemon juice
- Salt and pepper to taste

Directions:

1. In a bowl, combine the shredded carrots, diced red bell pepper, diced cucumber, diced red onion, chopped spinach, lemon juice, salt, and pepper. Toss to mix well.

2. Lay out one whole wheat tortilla on a clean, flat surface.

3. Spread a generous 1.4 oz (40 g) layer of hummus evenly over the entire tortilla.

4. Spoon the vegetable mixture evenly over the hummus layer.

5. Starting from the bottom edge of the tortilla, tightly roll it up, encasing the vegetables and hummus in a cylinder shape.

6. Use a sharp knife to slice the rolled tortilla into pinwheel-sized pieces, about 1 inch (2.5 cm) thick.

7. Repeat the process with the remaining tortillas.

8. Serve your carrot and hummus pinwheels as a delightful snack or appetizer.

Useful Tip: To make the tortillas easier to roll, you can warm them slightly in the microwave or on a griddle before assembling the pinwheels.

Nutritional Values: Calories: 190 kcal | Fat: 7 g | Protein: 6 g | Carbs: 27 g | Net carbs: 21 g | Fiber: 6 g | Cholesterol: 0 mg | Sodium: 370 mg | Potassium: 240 mg

Pear and Almond Butter Sandwiches

Serving: 4 | **Prep time:** 10 minutes | **Cook time:** 0 minutes

Ingredients:

- 8 slices of whole-grain bread
- 3.5 oz (100 g) almond butter
- 2 ripe pears, thinly sliced (about 14 oz or 400 g)
- 1.4 oz (40 g) honey
- 0.7 oz (20 g) chopped almonds
- 0.7 oz (20 g) dried cranberries
- Ground cinnamon, to taste

Directions:

1. Lay out 8 slices of whole-grain bread on a clean surface.
2. Spread a generous amount (about 0.4 oz or 12 g) of almond butter onto one side of each slice of bread.
3. Place thinly sliced ripe pear over the almond butter on 4 of the bread slices.
4. Drizzle honey evenly over the pear slices on each of the 4 slices.
5. Sprinkle chopped almonds and dried cranberries over the pear and honey.
6. Sprinkle ground cinnamon to taste over the almond butter on the remaining 4 slices of bread.
7. Carefully place the cinnamon-covered slices onto the almond butter, creating 4 sandwiches.
8. Gently press down on each sandwich to help the ingredients stick together.
9. Use a sharp knife to cut each sandwich into halves or quarters, depending on your preference.
10. Serve your pear and almond butter sandwiches as a delicious and healthy snack or light meal.

Useful Tip: If you want a warm sandwich, you can lightly toast the bread slices before assembling the sandwiches.

Nutritional Values: Calories: 320 kcal | Fat: 14 g | Protein: 8 g | Carbs: 42 g | Net carbs: 30 g | Fiber: 6 g | Cholesterol: 0 mg | Sodium: 240 mg | Potassium: 310 mg

Rice Cake with Avocado and Tomato

Serving: 4 | Prep time: 10 minutes | Cook time: 0 minutes

Ingredients:

- 4 rice cakes (about 2.8 oz or 80 g)
- 1 ripe avocado, sliced (about 7 oz or 200 g)
- 2 medium tomatoes, sliced (about 10.6 oz or 300 g)
- 1.4 oz (40 g) fresh basil leaves
- 1.4 oz (40 g) feta cheese, crumbled
- 1.4 oz (40 g) balsamic glaze
- Salt and pepper, to taste

Directions:

1. Lay out 4 rice cakes on a clean surface.
2. Place sliced avocado on each rice cake.
3. Top the avocado with tomato slices.
4. Sprinkle fresh basil leaves evenly over the tomato slices.
5. Crumble feta cheese and distribute it over the basil leaves.
6. Drizzle balsamic glaze over each rice cake, creating a flavorful dressing.
7. Season with a pinch of salt and pepper to taste.
8. Your rice cakes with avocado and tomato are ready to serve.

Useful Tip: You can add a protein boost by placing a grilled chicken breast or tofu slice on each rice cake before adding the avocado and tomato.

Nutritional Values: Calories: 190 kcal | Fat: 10 g | Protein: 3 g | Carbs: 24 g | Net carbs: 16 g | Fiber: 8 g | Cholesterol: 5 mg | Sodium: 180 mg | Potassium: 510 mg

Cantaloupe and Prosciutto Skewers

Serving: 4 | Prep time: 15 minutes | Cook time: 0 minutes

Ingredients:

- 1 small cantaloupe (about 2.2 lbs or 1 kg), peeled, seeded, and cut into bite-sized pieces
- 6 oz (170 g) prosciutto, thinly sliced
- 1.4 oz (40 g) fresh basil leaves
- Wooden skewers (soaked in water for 30 minutes to prevent splintering)
- 1.4 oz (40 ml)Balsamic glaze for drizzling
- Freshly ground black pepper, to taste

Directions:

1. Take a piece of cantaloupe and fold a slice of prosciutto around it.
2. Thread the cantaloupe and prosciutto bundle onto a wooden skewer.
3. Repeat this process for the remaining cantaloupe and prosciutto slices.
4. Slide a fresh basil leaf onto each skewer between the cantaloupe and prosciutto bundles.
5. Arrange the skewers on a serving platter.
6. Drizzle balsamic glaze over the skewers, and sprinkle freshly ground black pepper on top.
7. Your Cantaloupe and Prosciutto Skewers are ready to delight your taste buds.

Useful Tip: You can customize these skewers by adding small mozzarella balls (bocconcini) or cherry tomatoes for extra flavor and color.

Nutritional Values: Calories: 145 kcal | Fat: 6 g | Protein: 6 g | Carbs: 16 g | Net carbs: 14 g | Fiber: 2 g | Cholesterol: 20 mg | Sodium: 950 mg | Potassium: 430 mg

Tomato and Basil Bruschetta

Serving: 4 | Prep time: 10 minutes | Cook time: 5 minutes

Ingredients:

- 4 large ripe tomatoes (about 1.5 lbs or 680 g), finely diced
- 2.5 oz (70 g) fresh basil leaves, finely chopped
- 2 cloves garlic, minced
- 2.5 oz (70 g) red onion, finely diced
- 1 oz (28 g) extra-virgin olive oil
- 1 oz (28 g) balsamic vinegar
- Salt and freshly ground black pepper, to taste
- 8 slices of whole-grain bread, toasted

Directions:

1. In a large bowl, combine the diced tomatoes, minced garlic, finely chopped basil, and finely diced red onion.
2. Drizzle extra-virgin olive oil and balsamic vinegar over the tomato mixture.
3. Season with salt and freshly ground black pepper to taste. Mix well.
4. Let the tomato mixture sit for about 10 minutes to allow the flavors to meld.
5. While the mixture is resting, toast the slices of whole-grain bread until they are crispy.
6. Spoon the tomato and basil mixture generously over each toasted bread slice.
7. Serve immediately, and savor the fresh flavors of Tomato and Basil Bruschetta.

Useful Tip: For added creaminess, you can spread a thin layer of ricotta cheese on the toasted bread slices before adding the tomato and basil mixture.

Nutritional Values: Calories: 230 kcal | Fat: 10 g | Protein: 5 g | Carbs: 30 g | Net carbs: 21 g | Fiber: 9 g | Cholesterol: 0 mg | Sodium: 250 mg | Potassium: 540 mg

Pineapple and Cottage Cheese Bowls

Serving: 4 | Prep time: 15 minutes | Cook time: 0 minutes

Ingredients:

- 16 oz (450 g) fresh pineapple, diced
- 16 oz (450 g) low-fat cottage cheese
- 1.5 oz (42 g) honey
- 1.5 oz (42 g) chopped walnuts
- 1.5 oz (42 g) dried cranberries
- 1 tsp vanilla extract
- Fresh mint leaves for garnish (optional)

Directions:

1. In a mixing bowl, combine the low-fat cottage cheese and vanilla extract, and mix well.
2. In another bowl, combine the diced fresh pineapple, chopped walnuts, and dried cranberries.
3. Drizzle honey over the pineapple mixture and gently toss to combine.
4. To assemble each bowl, start with a scoop of the vanilla-flavored cottage cheese.
5. Top the cottage cheese with the sweet and tangy pineapple mixture.
6. Garnish with fresh mint leaves if desired.
7. Serve immediately and enjoy these refreshing Pineapple and Cottage Cheese Bowls.

Useful Tip: You can refrigerate the cottage cheese mixture and pineapple mixture separately in airtight containers and assemble the bowls just before serving for a chilled and refreshing treat.

Nutritional Values: Calories: 230 kcal | Fat: 7 g | Protein: 15 g | Carbs: 30 g | Net carbs: 24 g | Fiber: 6 g | Cholesterol: 10 mg | Sodium: 350 mg | Potassium: 330 mg

FISH AND SEAFOOD RECIPES

Baked Lemon Herb Salmon

Serving: 4 | Prep time: 10 minutes | Cook time: 15 minutes

Ingredients:

- 4 salmon fillets (4 oz / 113 g each)
- 1 lemon, thinly sliced
- 2 cloves garlic, minced
- 2 tbsp olive oil
- 1 tsp fresh lemon juice
- 1 tsp fresh thyme leaves
- 1 tsp fresh rosemary leaves, chopped
- Salt and pepper to taste
- Fresh parsley for garnish

Directions:

1. Preheat your oven to 375°F (190°C).
2. Place the salmon fillets on a baking sheet lined with parchment paper.
3. In a small bowl, whisk together the olive oil, minced garlic, fresh lemon juice, thyme, rosemary, salt, and pepper.
4. Brush the olive oil and herb mixture evenly over each salmon fillet.
5. Lay the lemon slices on top of the salmon fillets.
6. Bake in the preheated oven for about 15 minutes or until the salmon flakes easily with a fork.
7. Garnish with fresh parsley before serving.

Useful Tip: For an extra burst of flavor, marinate the salmon fillets in the olive oil and herb mixture for 30 minutes in the refrigerator before baking.

Nutritional Values: Calories: 250 kcal | Fat: 15 g | Protein: 25 g | Carbs: 2 g | Net carbs: 1 g | Fiber: 1 g | Cholesterol: 70 mg | Sodium: 80 mg | Potassium: 570 mg

Grilled Shrimp Skewers

Serving: 4 | Prep time: 20 minutes | Cook time: 6-8 minutes

Ingredients:

- 16 large shrimp, peeled and deveined (16 oz / 450 g)
- 2 cloves garlic, minced
- 2 tbsp olive oil
- 1 tsp fresh lemon juice
- 1 tsp fresh parsley, chopped
- 1/2 tsp smoked paprika
- 1/2 tsp cayenne pepper (adjust to taste)
- Salt and pepper to taste
- Wooden skewers, soaked in water for 30 minutes
- Lemon wedges for garnish

Directions:

1. In a bowl, combine the minced garlic, olive oil, fresh lemon juice, chopped parsley, smoked paprika, cayenne pepper, salt, and pepper.
2. Thread four shrimp onto each soaked wooden skewer.
3. Brush the shrimp skewers with the garlic and herb mixture, ensuring they are evenly coated.
4. Preheat your grill to medium-high heat (about 400°F / 200°C).
5. Place the shrimp skewers on the grill and cook for 2-4 minutes per side, or until they turn pink and opaque. Be careful not to overcook, as shrimp can become tough.
6. Remove the skewers from the grill and garnish with lemon wedges.

Useful Tip: For extra flavor, you can marinate the shrimp in the garlic and herb mixture for 15-20 minutes before grilling.

Nutritional Values: Calories: 150 kcal | Fat: 8 g | Protein: 18 g | Carbs: 2 g | Net carbs: 1 g | Fiber: 1 g | Cholesterol: 180 mg | Sodium: 220 mg | Potassium: 180 mg

Baked Cod with Tomato and Basil

Serving: 4 | Prep time: 15 minutes | Cook time: 20 minutes

Ingredients:

- 4 cod fillets (4 oz / 115 g each)
- 2 tomatoes, diced (8 oz / 225 g)
- 2 tbsp fresh basil leaves, chopped
- 2 cloves garlic, minced
- 2 tbsp olive oil
- 1 tbsp balsamic vinegar
- Salt and pepper to taste
- Lemon wedges for garnish

Directions:

1. Preheat your oven to 375°F (190°C).
2. In a bowl, combine the diced tomatoes, chopped basil, minced garlic, olive oil, balsamic vinegar, salt, and pepper. Mix well to create the tomato and basil salsa.
3. Place the cod fillets in a baking dish and season them with a pinch of salt and pepper.
4. Spoon the tomato and basil salsa evenly over the cod fillets.
5. Cover the baking dish with aluminum foil and bake in the preheated oven for 15-20 minutes, or until the cod is cooked through and flakes easily with a fork.
6. Remove the foil and broil for an additional 2-3 minutes, or until the top is slightly browned.
7. Garnish with lemon wedges before serving.

Useful Tip: You can substitute cod with other white fish such as haddock or tilapia if desired.

Nutritional Values: Calories: 220 kcal | Fat: 9 g | Protein: 27 g | Carbs: 6 g | Net carbs: 4 g | Fiber: 2 g | Cholesterol: 60 mg | Sodium: 160 mg | Potassium: 720 mg

Lemon Garlic Butter Scallops

Serving: 4 | Prep time: 10 minutes | Cook time: 5 minutes

Ingredients:

- 16 large sea scallops (16 oz / 450 g)
- 2 tbsp olive oil
- 3 cloves garlic, minced
- 2 tbsp unsalted butter
- Zest and juice of 1 lemon
- Salt and pepper to taste
- Fresh parsley, chopped, for garnish

Directions:

1. Pat the scallops dry with paper towels to remove excess moisture. Season both sides with a pinch of salt and pepper.
2. Heat olive oil in a large skillet over medium-high heat.
3. Add the scallops to the hot skillet and sear for 1-2 minutes on each side, or until they develop a golden crust and are just cooked through. Remove them from the skillet and set aside.
4. In the same skillet, add minced garlic and cook for about 30 seconds until fragrant, being careful not to burn it.
5. Reduce the heat to medium-low and add the unsalted butter, lemon zest, lemon juice. Stir well to combine and allow the sauce to simmer for 2-3 minutes, reducing slightly.
6. Return the seared scallops to the skillet and coat them with the lemon garlic butter sauce for an additional 1-2 minutes, or until they are heated through.
7. Serve the scallops immediately, garnished with freshly chopped parsley.

Useful Tip: Be cautious not to overcook the scallops, as they can become tough. They should be opaque and slightly translucent in the center when done.

Nutritional Values: Calories: 240 kcal | Fat: 11 g | Protein: 23 g | Carbs: 6 g | Net carbs: 4 g | Fiber: 2 g | Cholesterol: 60 mg | Sodium: 570 mg | Potassium: 370 mg

Poached Tilapia with Herbed Yogurt

Serving: 4 | Prep time: 10 minutes | Cook time: 15 minutes

Ingredients:

- 16 oz (450 g) tilapia fillets (4 fillets)
- 16 oz (480 ml) low-sodium chicken broth
- 1 lemon, thinly sliced
- 1 bay leaf
- 4 oz (120 g) Greek yogurt
- 0.5 oz (15 ml) olive oil
- 0.5 oz (15 g) garlic, minced
- 0.25 oz (15 g) fresh dill, chopped
- 0.25 oz (15 g) fresh parsley, chopped
- Salt and pepper to taste
- Lemon wedges, for garnish

Directions:

1. In a large skillet or shallow pan, combine the low-sodium chicken broth, lemon slices, and bay leaf. Bring the mixture to a gentle simmer over medium heat.

2. Carefully place the tilapia fillets into the simmering broth. Poach them for about 6-8 minutes, or until the fish is opaque and flakes easily with a fork.

3. While the tilapia is poaching, prepare the herbed yogurt. In a small mixing bowl, combine the Greek yogurt, olive oil, minced garlic, chopped dill, and chopped parsley. Season with a pinch of salt and pepper. Mix until well combined.

4. Once the tilapia is done, use a slotted spoon to remove the fillets from the poaching liquid, allowing any excess liquid to drain.

5. Serve the poached tilapia fillets with a generous dollop of herbed yogurt on top. Garnish with lemon wedges for added flavor.

Useful Tip: You can customize the herbed yogurt with your favorite fresh herbs, such as cilantro or chives, for a different flavor profile.

Nutritional Values: Calories: 220 kcal | Fat: 7 g | Protein: 32 g | Carbs: 6 g | Net carbs: 4 g | Fiber: 2 g | Cholesterol: 70 mg | Sodium: 320 mg | Potassium: 650 mg

Salmon and Asparagus Foil Packets

Serving: 4 | Prep time: 10 minutes | Cook time: 20 minutes

Ingredients:

- 16 oz (450 g) salmon fillets (4 fillets)
- 16 oz (450 g) asparagus spears (16 spears)
- 2 oz (60 ml) olive oil
- 0.5 oz (15 g) garlic, minced
- 1 lemon, thinly sliced
- 0.25 oz (7 g) fresh dill, chopped
- Salt and pepper to taste
- 4 sheets of aluminum foil (about 12x18 inches each)

Directions:

1. Preheat your oven to 400°F (200°C).

2. Place each salmon fillet on a separate sheet of aluminum foil. Season the salmon with minced garlic, salt, and pepper.

3. Lay 4 asparagus spears on top of each salmon fillet.

4. Drizzle olive oil over each salmon and asparagus stack.

5. Add a couple of lemon slices on top of each stack, and sprinkle fresh dill over them.

6. Fold the aluminum foil over the salmon and asparagus, creating a packet. Ensure it's sealed tightly to trap the steam.

7. Place the foil packets on a baking sheet and bake in the preheated oven for about 15-20 minutes, or until the salmon flakes easily with a fork and the asparagus is tender.

8. Carefully open the foil packets, and serve the salmon and asparagus right from the packets.

Useful Tip: You can customize these foil packets with your favorite herbs and seasonings, such as adding a pinch of paprika or substituting dill with thyme for a different flavor profile.

Nutritional Values: Calories: 350 kcal | Fat: 23 g | Protein: 30 g | Carbs: 7 g | Net carbs: 4 g | Fiber: 3 g | Cholesterol: 75 mg | Sodium: 150 mg | Potassium: 950 mg

Lime Cilantro Shrimp Tacos

Serving: 4 | Prep time: 15 minutes | Cook time: 10 minutes

Ingredients:

- 16 oz (450 g) large shrimp, peeled and deveined
- 2 oz (60 ml) lime juice (about 2 limes)
- 1 oz (30 g) fresh cilantro, chopped
- 1 oz (30 ml) olive oil
- 2 cloves garlic, minced
- 1 tsp honey
- 0.25 oz (7 g) chili powder
- Salt and pepper to taste
- 8 small corn tortillas
- 4 oz (140 g) shredded lettuce
- 4 oz (150 g) diced tomatoes
- 2 oz (60 g) diced red onion
- 2 oz (30 g) crumbled queso fresco (optional)
- Lime wedges for garnish

Directions:

1. In a bowl, combine the lime juice, chopped cilantro, olive oil, minced garlic, honey, chili powder, salt, and pepper to create the marinade.

2. Place the peeled and deveined shrimp in a resealable plastic bag and pour the marinade over them. Seal the bag and shake it gently to coat the shrimp. Marinate in the refrigerator for at least 15 minutes.

3. Preheat a grill or skillet over medium-high heat. Thread the marinated shrimp onto skewers if using a grill, or you can cook them directly in a skillet.

4. Grill or cook the shrimp for about 2-3 minutes per side or until they turn pink and opaque.

5. While the shrimp are cooking, warm the corn tortillas in the oven or on the stovetop.

6. To assemble the tacos, place a few shrimp on each tortilla. Top with shredded lettuce, diced tomatoes, diced red onion, and crumbled queso fresco if desired.

7. Garnish with additional fresh cilantro and serve with lime wedges on the side.

Useful Tip: To add an extra kick to your tacos, consider making a quick lime crema by mixing some lime juice and sour cream or Greek yogurt.

Nutritional Values: Calories: 280 kcal | Fat: 8 g | Protein: 24 g | Carbs: 28 g | Net carbs: 20 g | Fiber: 8 g | Cholesterol: 180 mg | Sodium: 270 mg | Potassium: 460 mg

Lime Herb-Crusted Halibut

Serving: 4 | Prep time: 10 minutes | Cook time: 15 minutes

Ingredients:

- 16 oz (450 g) halibut fillets (four 4 oz fillets)
- 1 oz (30 ml) lime juice (about 2 limes)
- 2 oz (60 g) almond flour
- 0.5 oz (15 g) fresh parsley, finely chopped
- 0.5 oz (15 g) fresh cilantro, finely chopped
- 1 oz (30 ml) olive oil
- 2 cloves garlic, minced
- 0.25 oz (7 g) ground flaxseed
- Salt and pepper to taste
- Lime wedges for garnish

Directions:

1. Preheat your oven to 375°F (190°C).

2. In a bowl, combine the almond flour, finely chopped parsley, finely chopped cilantro, minced garlic, ground flaxseed, salt, and pepper. Mix well to create the herb crust.

3. Drizzle the lime juice over the halibut fillets to give them a citrusy flavor.

4. Place the herb crust mixture on a plate. Coat each halibut fillet with the herb crust mixture, pressing it onto the fillets to adhere.

5. In an oven-safe skillet, heat the olive oil over medium-high heat. Once hot, add the herb-crusted halibut fillets to the skillet.

6. Sear the fillets for about 2-3 minutes on each side until they develop a golden crust.

7. Transfer the skillet to the preheated oven and bake for an additional 5-7 minutes or until the halibut is cooked through and flakes easily with a fork.

8. Garnish the halibut with lime wedges before serving.

Useful Tip: To check if the halibut is cooked, insert a fork into the thickest part of the fillet. It should flake easily and be opaque throughout.

Nutritional Values: Calories: 300 kcal | Fat: 19 g | Protein: 26 g | Carbs: 8 g | Net carbs: 4 g | Fiber: 4 g | Cholesterol: 55 mg | Sodium: 250 mg | Potassium: 620 mg

Baked Teriyaki Salmon

Serving: 4 | Prep time: 15 minutes | Cook time: 20 minutes

Ingredients:

- 16 oz (450 g) salmon fillets (four 4 oz fillets)
- 2 oz (60 ml) low-sodium soy sauce
- 1 oz (30 ml) water
- 2 oz (60 ml) rice vinegar
- 1 oz (30 ml) honey
- 2 cloves garlic, minced
- 1 oz (30 g) fresh ginger, grated
- 0.5 oz (15 g) sesame seeds
- 0.5 oz (15 g) green onions, thinly sliced
- Salt and pepper to taste
- Cooking spray

Directions:

1. Preheat your oven to 375°F (190°C).

2. In a saucepan over medium heat, combine the low-sodium soy sauce, water, rice vinegar, honey, minced garlic, and grated ginger. Stir well and simmer for about 5-7 minutes until the sauce thickens slightly.

3. Place the salmon fillets on a baking sheet lined with parchment paper. Season them with salt and pepper to taste.

4. Pour half of the teriyaki sauce over the salmon fillets, making sure to coat them evenly.

5. Bake the salmon in the preheated oven for 15-18 minutes or until the salmon flakes easily with a fork and reaches your desired level of doneness.

6. While the salmon is baking, toast the sesame seeds in a dry skillet over medium heat until they turn golden brown. Set them aside.

7. Once the salmon is done, drizzle the remaining teriyaki sauce over the top.

8. Sprinkle the toasted sesame seeds and thinly sliced green onions over the salmon as a garnish.

Useful Tip: To prevent the salmon from sticking to the parchment paper, lightly spray the paper with cooking spray before placing the fillets on it.

Nutritional Values: Calories: 300 kcal | Fat: 10 g | Protein: 26 g | Carbs: 20 g | Net carbs: 18 g | Fiber: 2 g | Cholesterol: 65 mg | Sodium: 500 mg | Potassium: 600 mg

Seared Scallops with Mango Salsa

Serving: 4 | Prep time: 15 minutes | Cook time: 10 minutes

Ingredients:

- 16 large sea scallops (about 16 oz or 450 g)
- 2 oz (60 ml) olive oil, divided
- Salt and black pepper to taste
- 2 ripe mangoes, peeled, pitted, and diced (about 16 oz or 450 g)
- 1 small red onion, finely chopped (about 2 oz or 60 g)
- 1 red bell pepper, diced (about 4 oz or 120 g)
- 1 jalapeño pepper, seeded and finely chopped (adjust to your preferred spice level)
- 2 oz (60 ml) fresh lime juice
- 0.5 oz (15 g) fresh cilantro, chopped
- 1 oz (30 g) fresh mint leaves, chopped

Directions:

1. Start by making the mango salsa. In a bowl, combine the diced mangoes, finely chopped red onion, diced red bell pepper, chopped jalapeño pepper, fresh lime juice, chopped cilantro, and chopped mint leaves. Mix well, and season with salt and pepper to taste. Refrigerate the salsa to let the flavors meld while you prepare the scallops.

2. Pat the scallops dry with paper towels to remove excess moisture, which will help them sear better.

3. Season the scallops with salt and black pepper on both sides.

4. Heat 1 oz (30 ml) of olive oil in a large skillet over high heat until it begins to shimmer.

5. Carefully add the seasoned scallops to the hot skillet, ensuring they are not overcrowded. Sear the scallops for about 2-3 minutes on each side, or until they develop a golden-brown crust and are opaque in the center. Be careful not to overcook; scallops should be tender.

6. While searing, drizzle the remaining 1 oz (30 ml) of olive oil over the scallops to enhance their flavor.

7. Once the scallops are seared to perfection, remove them from the skillet.

8. To serve, place a generous spoonful of the mango salsa on each plate and top with seared scallops.

Useful Tip: For the best sear on scallops, make sure they are completely dry before cooking and avoid overcrowding the pan.

Nutritional Values: Calories: 300 kcal | Fat: 10 g | Protein: 20 g | Carbs: 30 g | Net carbs: 22 g | Fiber: 8 g | Cholesterol: 35 mg | Sodium: 500 mg | Potassium: 750 mg

Broiled Lemon Pepper Haddock

Serving: 4 | Prep time: 10 minutes | Cook time: 10 minutes

Ingredients:

- 4 haddock fillets (about 16 oz or 450 g)
- 1 oz (30 ml) olive oil
- 1 lemon, juiced and zested
- 1 tsp black pepper
- 1/2 tsp garlic powder
- 1/2 tsp onion powder
- 1/2 tsp dried thyme
- 1/2 tsp dried oregano
- 1/2 tsp dried basil
- 1/2 tsp dried parsley
- 1/2 tsp paprika
- Salt to taste
- Lemon wedges for garnish

Directions:

1. Preheat your broiler to high and adjust the oven rack to the top position.

2. In a small bowl, combine the olive oil, lemon juice, lemon zest, black pepper, garlic powder, onion powder, dried thyme, dried oregano, dried basil, dried parsley, paprika, and a pinch of salt. Mix well to create a flavorful marinade.

3. Place the haddock fillets on a baking sheet lined with aluminum foil for easy cleanup.

4. Brush the marinade generously over the haddock fillets, ensuring they are well-coated on both sides.

5. Place the baking sheet with the marinated haddock under the broiler and cook for approximately 4-5 minutes on each side or until the fish flakes easily with a fork and has a beautiful golden color.

6. Remove the haddock from the broiler and garnish with lemon wedges.

Useful Tip: When broiling, keep a close eye on the fish as it can cook quickly. Overcooking can make the fish dry, so it's best to check for doneness by using a fork to see if it flakes easily.

Nutritional Values: Calories: 220 kcal | Fat: 9 g | Protein: 30 g | Carbs: 4 g | Net carbs: 2 g | Fiber: 2 g | Cholesterol: 75 mg | Sodium: 200 mg | Potassium: 600 mg

Shrimp and Vegetable Stir-Fry

Serving: 4 | Prep time: 15 minutes | Cook time: 10 minutes

Ingredients:

- 16 oz (450 g) large shrimp, peeled and deveined
- 8 oz (225 g) broccoli florets
- 4 oz (115 g) snap peas, trimmed
- 1 red bell pepper, thinly sliced
- 1 yellow bell pepper, thinly sliced
- 1 medium carrot, julienned
- 2 cloves garlic, minced
- 1-inch (2.5 cm) piece of fresh ginger, minced
- 2 tbsp low-sodium soy sauce
- 1 tbsp sesame oil
- 1 tsp rice vinegar
- 1/2 tsp honey or a low-calorie sweetener of your choice
- 1/2 tsp cornstarch
- 1/4 tsp crushed red pepper flakes (adjust to taste)
- 1 tbsp vegetable oil for stir-frying
- Salt and pepper to taste
- Fresh cilantro leaves for garnish
- Cooked brown rice for serving (optional)

Directions:

1. In a small bowl, whisk together the soy sauce, sesame oil, rice vinegar, honey (or sweetener), cornstarch, and crushed red pepper flakes. Set this sauce aside.

2. Heat the vegetable oil in a large skillet or wok over medium-high heat. Add the minced garlic and ginger, and stir-fry for about 30 seconds until fragrant.

3. Add the shrimp to the skillet and cook for 2-3 minutes on each side or until they turn pink and opaque. Remove the cooked shrimp from the skillet and set them aside.

4. In the same skillet, add a bit more vegetable oil if needed. Add the broccoli, snap peas, bell pepper and julienned carrots. Stir-fry the vegetables for about 3-4 minutes or until they become tender-crisp.

5. Return the cooked shrimp to the skillet and pour the sauce over the shrimp and vegetables. Toss everything together and cook for an additional 2-3 minutes until the sauce thickens and coats the ingredients evenly.

6. Season with salt and pepper to taste.

7. Serve the shrimp and vegetable stir-fry over cooked brown rice if desired, and garnish with fresh cilantro leaves.

Useful Tip: To save time on busy weeknights, you can prep and chop all your ingredients in advance, so they're ready to go when it's time to stir-fry.

Nutritional Values: Calories: 190 kcal | Fat: 5 g | Protein: 24 g | Carbs: 15 g | Net carbs: 9 g | Fiber: 6 g | Cholesterol: 170 mg | Sodium: 450 mg | Potassium: 640 mg

Baked Coconut-Crusted Tilapia

Serving: 4 | Prep time: 15 minutes | Cook time: 15 minutes

Ingredients:

- 4 tilapia fillets (4 oz or 115 g each)
- 2 oz (55 g) unsweetened shredded coconut
- 2 oz (55 g) almond meal
- 1 tsp paprika
- 1/2 tsp garlic powder
- 1/2 tsp onion powder
- 1/4 tsp cayenne pepper (adjust to taste)
- 2 large eggs, beaten
- 1 tbsp olive oil
- Salt and pepper to taste
- Lemon wedges for serving

Directions:

1. Preheat your oven to 375°F (190°C) and line a baking sheet with parchment paper.
2. In a shallow dish, combine the unsweetened shredded coconut, almond meal, paprika, garlic powder, onion powder, and cayenne pepper. Mix well.
3. Season the tilapia fillets with salt and pepper.
4. Dip each tilapia fillet into the beaten eggs, allowing any excess to drip off.
5. Coat the fillets in the coconut and almond mixture, pressing gently to adhere the coating to the fish.
6. Place the coated tilapia fillets on the prepared baking sheet.
7. Drizzle each fillet with a bit of olive oil to help the coating turn golden brown.
8. Bake in the preheated oven for 12-15 minutes or until the fish is opaque and easily flakes with a fork.
9. Serve the baked coconut-crusted tilapia with lemon wedges for a zesty touch.

Useful Tip: To ensure a crispier crust, you can briefly broil the tilapia under a high broiler for 1-2 minutes after baking.

Nutritional Values: Calories: 290 kcal | Fat: 18 g | Protein: 25 g | Carbs: 8 g | Net carbs: 4 g | Fiber: 4 g | Cholesterol: 145 mg | Sodium: 140 mg | Potassium: 340 mg

Salmon and Spinach Stuffed Mushrooms

Serving: 4 | Prep time: 20 minutes | Cook time: 20 minutes

Ingredients:

- 16 large mushrooms, cleaned and stems removed
- 8 oz (225 g) salmon fillet, cooked and flaked
- 4 oz (115 g) fresh spinach, chopped
- 2 oz (55 g) cream cheese
- 2 oz (60 ml) grated Parmesan cheese
- 2 cloves garlic, minced
- 1 tsp olive oil
- 1/2 tsp dried dill
- Salt and pepper to taste
- Fresh dill or parsley for garnish

Directions:

1. Preheat your oven to 375°F (190°C) and line a baking sheet with parchment paper.
2. In a skillet, heat the olive oil over medium heat. Add the minced garlic and cook for about 1 minute until fragrant.
3. Add the chopped spinach to the skillet and sauté for 2-3 minutes until it wilts. Remove from heat.
4. In a mixing bowl, combine the flaked salmon, sautéed spinach, cream cheese, grated Parmesan, dried dill, salt, and pepper. Mix until well combined.
5. Take each mushroom cap and fill it generously with the salmon and spinach mixture, packing it down slightly.
6. Arrange the stuffed mushrooms on the prepared baking sheet.
7. Bake in the preheated oven for about 15-20 minutes or until the mushrooms are tender and the filling is

golden brown.

8. Garnish with fresh dill or parsley before serving.

Useful Tip: You can add a squeeze of fresh lemon juice over the stuffed mushrooms just before serving for a burst of citrus flavor.

Nutritional Values: Calories: 170 kcal | Fat: 9 g | Protein: 15 g | Carbs: 7 g | Net carbs: 3 g | Fiber: 4 g | Cholesterol: 45 mg | Sodium: 210 mg | Potassium: 720 mg

Cilantro Lime Grilled Swordfish

Serving: 4 | Prep time: 15 minutes | Cook time: 10 minutes

Ingredients:

- 4 swordfish steaks, 6 oz (170 g) each
- 2 oz (60 ml) fresh lime juice
- 2 tbsp olive oil
- 2 cloves garlic, minced

- 0.5 oz (15 g) fresh cilantro, chopped
- 1 tsp ground cumin
- Salt and pepper to taste
- Lime wedges for garnish

Directions:

1. In a small bowl, whisk together the fresh lime juice, olive oil, minced garlic, chopped cilantro, ground cumin, salt, and pepper to create the marinade.
2. Place the swordfish steaks in a shallow dish and pour the marinade over them. Make sure each steak is well coated. Cover and refrigerate for at least 15 minutes, allowing the flavors to meld.
3. Preheat your grill to medium-high heat (about 400°F or 200°C). Make sure the grates are clean and lightly oiled to prevent sticking.
4. Remove the swordfish steaks from the marinade and let any excess marinade drip off.
5. Grill the swordfish steaks for about 4-5 minutes per side, or until they are opaque and easily flake with a fork. Cooking time may vary depending on the thickness of the steaks.
6. While grilling, you can brush some of the leftover marinade onto the swordfish for extra flavor.
7. Once done, transfer the grilled swordfish steaks to a serving platter.
8. Garnish with lime wedges and additional fresh cilantro if desired.

Useful Tip: Swordfish is dense and meaty, so it's essential not to overcook it to keep it tender and juicy. Use a meat thermometer to ensure the internal temperature reaches 145°F (63°C).

Nutritional Values: Calories: 300 kcal | Fat: 14 g | Protein: 36 g | Carbs: 3 g | Net carbs: 2 g | Fiber: 1 g | Cholesterol: 75 mg | Sodium: 220 mg | Potassium: 820 mg

Baked Garlic Herb Mussels

Serving: 4 | Prep time: 15 minutes | Cook time: 12 minutes

Ingredients:

- 32 fresh mussels, cleaned and debearded (about 2 lbs or 900 g)
- 2 oz (60 ml) chicken or vegetable broth
- 2 cloves garlic, minced
- 1 oz (30 g) fresh parsley, chopped

- 1 oz (30 g) fresh chives, chopped
- 2 oz (60 g) unsalted butter, melted
- Salt and pepper to taste
- Lemon wedges for garnish

Directions:

1. Preheat your oven to 425°F (220°C).
2. In a large ovenproof skillet or baking dish, combine the chicken or vegetable broth.
3. Place the cleaned mussels into the skillet in a single layer.
4. Sprinkle the minced garlic, fresh parsley, and fresh chives over the mussels.

5. Drizzle the melted unsalted butter evenly over the mussels, and season with salt and pepper to taste.

6. Cover the skillet with a lid or aluminum foil and bake in the preheated oven for about 10-12 minutes or until the mussels have opened and are cooked through. Discard any mussels that remain closed.

7. Once done, remove the skillet from the oven.

8. Serve the baked garlic herb mussels hot, garnished with lemon wedges.

Useful Tip: Before baking, give the skillet a gentle shake to distribute the flavors and ensure even cooking.

Nutritional Values: Calories: 280 kcal | Fat: 16 g | Protein: 21 g | Carbs: 8 g | Net carbs: 6 g | Fiber: 2 g | Cholesterol: 85 mg | Sodium: 580 mg | Potassium: 500 mg

Herb-Crusted Mahi-Mahi

Serving: 4 | Prep time: 10 minutes | Cook time: 15 minutes

Ingredients:

- 4 Mahi-Mahi fillets (about 6 oz or 170 g each)
- 2 oz (60 g) fresh parsley, finely chopped
- 1 oz (30 g) fresh thyme leaves, stripped from stems
- 1 oz (30 g) fresh rosemary leaves, chopped
- 2 oz (60 g) almond flour
- 2 oz (60 g) grated Parmesan cheese
- 2 cloves garlic, minced
- Zest of 1 lemon
- 2 oz (60 ml) olive oil
- Salt and pepper to taste
- Lemon wedges for serving

Directions:

1. Preheat your oven to 375°F (190°C).

2. In a mixing bowl, combine the finely chopped fresh parsley, thyme leaves, chopped rosemary, almond flour, grated Parmesan cheese, minced garlic, lemon zest, and olive oil. Mix until you have a coarse, herb-infused mixture.

3. Season the Mahi-Mahi fillets with salt and pepper to taste.

4. Place the fillets on a baking sheet lined with parchment paper.

5. Press the herb mixture evenly onto the top of each Mahi-Mahi fillet, forming a flavorful crust.

6. Bake the fillets in the preheated oven for approximately 15 minutes or until the fish is opaque and easily flakes with a fork.

7. Once done, remove the Herb-Crusted Mahi-Mahi from the oven.

8. Serve the fillets hot, garnished with lemon wedges for an extra zesty touch.

Useful Tip: For a crispy crust, you can briefly broil the fillets for 1-2 minutes after baking, but be sure to watch them closely to prevent burning.

Nutritional Values: Calories: 350 kcal | Fat: 18 g | Protein: 34 g | Carbs: 10 g | Net carbs: 6 g | Fiber: 4 g | Cholesterol: 110 mg | Sodium: 250 mg | Potassium: 600 mg

Lemon Pepper Baked Snapper

Serving: 4 | Prep time: 10 minutes | Cook time: 15 minutes

Ingredients:

- 4 snapper fillets (about 6 oz or 170 g each)
- 2 oz (60 g) almond meal
- 2 oz (60 g) grated Parmesan cheese
- Zest of 2 lemons
- 2 tsp lemon juice
- 2 tsp olive oil
- 1 tsp black pepper
- 1/2 tsp salt
- 2 cloves garlic, minced
- Fresh parsley for garnish

Directions:

1. Preheat your oven to 375°F (190°C).

2. In a bowl, combine the almond meal, grated Parmesan cheese, lemon zest, black pepper, salt, and minced garlic.

3. In a separate bowl, mix together the lemon juice and olive oil.

4. Season the snapper fillets with a pinch of salt.

5. Brush each snapper fillet with the lemon juice and olive oil mixture.

6. Coat the fillets generously with the almond meal and Parmesan mixture, pressing it onto the fish to form a flavorful crust.

7. Place the coated snapper fillets on a baking sheet lined with parchment paper.

8. Bake in the preheated oven for approximately 15 minutes or until the snapper is opaque and flakes easily with a fork.

9. Garnish with fresh parsley before serving.

Useful Tip: To make the crust even crispier, you can briefly broil the fillets for 1-2 minutes after baking, but be vigilant to prevent overcooking.

Nutritional Values: Calories: 300 kcal | Fat: 15 g | Protein: 30 g | Carbs: 8 g | Net carbs: 4 g | Fiber: 4 g | Cholesterol: 80 mg | Sodium: 500 mg | Potassium: 520 mg

Herbed Sea Bass with Cherry Tomatoes

Serving: 4 | Prep time: 15 minutes | Cook time: 20 minutes

Ingredients:

- 4 sea bass fillets (about 6 oz or 170 g each)
- 12 oz (340 g) cherry tomatoes
- 2 oz (60 g) fresh basil leaves
- 2 oz (60 g) fresh parsley leaves
- 2 cloves garlic
- 2 oz (60 g) pine nuts
- 2 oz (60 g) grated Parmesan cheese
- 2 oz (60 g) olive oil
- Zest of 1 lemon
- Salt and black pepper to taste
- Lemon wedges for garnish

Directions:

1. Preheat your oven to 375°F (190°C).

2. In a food processor, combine the fresh basil, fresh parsley, garlic, pine nuts, grated Parmesan cheese, and olive oil. Blend until you have a smooth herb paste.

3. Season the sea bass fillets with a pinch of salt, black pepper, and the lemon zest.

4. Spread a generous layer of the herb paste on each sea bass fillet.

5. Place the cherry tomatoes in a baking dish and drizzle them with a bit of olive oil, salt, and black pepper.

6. Arrange the sea bass fillets on top of the cherry tomatoes in the baking dish.

7. Bake in the preheated oven for approximately 20 minutes or until the sea bass is cooked through, and the tomatoes are tender.

8. Garnish with lemon wedges before serving.

Useful Tip: If you prefer a crispier texture, you can broil the sea bass for the last 2-3 minutes, but keep an eye on it to avoid overcooking.

Nutritional Values: Calories: 350 kcal | Fat: 25 g | Protein: 30 g | Carbs: 8 g | Net carbs: 4 g | Fiber: 4 g | Cholesterol: 70 mg | Sodium: 350 mg | Potassium: 650 mg

POULTRY AND MEAT RECIPES

Lemon Herb Grilled Chicken Breast

Serving: 4 | Prep time: 10 minutes | Cook time: 15 minutes

Ingredients:

- 4 boneless, skinless chicken breasts (about 5 oz or 140 g each)
- 2 oz (60 g) olive oil
- Zest and juice of 1 lemon
- 2 cloves garlic, minced
- 2 tsp fresh thyme leaves
- 2 tsp fresh rosemary leaves
- Salt and black pepper to taste
- Lemon wedges for garnish

Directions:

1. In a bowl, whisk together the olive oil, lemon zest, lemon juice, minced garlic, fresh thyme leaves, and fresh rosemary leaves.
2. Season the chicken breasts with a pinch of salt and black pepper.
3. Place the chicken breasts in a resealable plastic bag and pour the marinade over them. Seal the bag and massage the marinade into the chicken, ensuring they are well coated. Refrigerate for at least 30 minutes (or up to 4 hours for more flavor).
4. Preheat your grill to medium-high heat, about 375-400°F (190-200°C).
5. Remove the chicken breasts from the marinade and let any excess marinade drip off.
6. Grill the chicken for about 6-7 minutes on each side or until the internal temperature reaches 165°F (74°C) and the chicken is cooked through with beautiful grill marks.
7. Transfer the grilled chicken to a serving platter, garnish with lemon wedges, and serve.

Useful Tip: To ensure even cooking, you can pound the chicken breasts to an even thickness before marinating.

Nutritional Values: Calories: 280 kcal | Fat: 15 g | Protein: 30 g | Carbs: 2 g | Net carbs: 1 g | Fiber: 1 g | Cholesterol: 80 mg | Sodium: 320 mg | Potassium: 440 mg

Stuffed Bell Peppers with Lean Ground Beef

Serving: 4 | Prep time: 20 minutes | Cook time: 45 minutes

Ingredients:

- 4 large bell peppers (red, green, or yellow)
- 12 oz (340 g) lean ground beef
- 1 small onion, finely chopped
- 2 cloves garlic, minced
- 2 oz (60 g) brown rice, cooked
- 4 oz (115 g) tomato sauce
- 1 tsp olive oil
- 1 tsp dried oregano
- 1 tsp dried basil
- Salt and black pepper to taste
- 2 oz (60 g) low-fat shredded mozzarella cheese
- Fresh basil leaves for garnish

Directions:

1. Preheat your oven to 350°F (175°C).
2. Cut the tops off the bell peppers and remove the seeds and membranes. Set aside.
3. In a large skillet, heat the olive oil over medium heat. Add the chopped onion and garlic, and sauté for 2-3 minutes until they become translucent.
4. Add the lean ground beef to the skillet and cook, breaking it apart with a spatula, until it's browned and cooked through. Drain any excess fat.
5. Stir in the cooked brown rice, tomato sauce, dried oregano, dried basil, salt, and black pepper. Cook for an additional 2-3 minutes until well combined.

6. Carefully stuff each bell pepper with the beef and rice mixture, packing it in tightly. Place the stuffed peppers in a baking dish.

7. Cover the baking dish with foil and bake in the preheated oven for 30 minutes.

8. Remove the foil and sprinkle the shredded mozzarella cheese over the tops of the peppers. Return the dish to the oven and bake for an additional 10-15 minutes, or until the cheese is melted and bubbly.

9. Garnish with fresh basil leaves before serving.

Useful Tip: You can use any color of bell pepper for this recipe, or mix and match for a colorful presentation.

Nutritional Values: Calories: 350 kcal | Fat: 11 g | Protein: 26 g | Carbs: 38 g | Net carbs: 32 g | Fiber: 6 g | Cholesterol: 60 mg | Sodium: 500 mg | Potassium: 840 mg

Herb-Crusted Chicken Thighs

Serving: 4 | Prep time: 15 minutes | Cook time: 25 minutes

Ingredients:

- 4 boneless, skinless chicken thighs (about 16 oz or 450 g)
- 1 oz (30 g) fresh parsley, finely chopped
- 1 oz (30 g) fresh basil, finely chopped
- 1 oz (30 g) fresh rosemary, finely chopped
- 2 oz (60 g) whole-grain mustard
- 1 oz (30 g) grated Parmesan cheese
- 1 oz (30 g) ground almonds
- 1 oz (30 ml) olive oil
- 1 oz (30 ml) lemon juice
- 1 tsp lemon zest
- Salt and black pepper to taste
- Cooking spray

Directions:

1. Preheat your oven to 375°F (190°C).

2. In a mixing bowl, combine the finely chopped parsley, basil, and rosemary. This is your herb mixture.

3. In a separate bowl, mix together the whole-grain mustard, grated Parmesan cheese, ground almonds, olive oil, lemon juice, lemon zest, salt, and black pepper. This creates your herb and mustard mixture.

4. Lay the chicken thighs on a clean surface and pat them dry with a paper towel.

5. Take each chicken thigh and generously coat it in the herb and mustard mixture, ensuring it's evenly covered.

6. Next, dip the coated chicken thighs into the herb mixture, pressing the herbs onto the surface to create a crust.

7. Place a wire rack on a baking sheet and lightly coat it with cooking spray. Arrange the herb-crusted chicken thighs on the wire rack.

8. Bake in the preheated oven for approximately 20-25 minutes or until the chicken reaches an internal temperature of 165°F (74°C) and the crust is golden brown and crispy.

Useful Tip: You can customize the herb mixture by adding your favorite herbs for extra flavor.

Nutritional Values: Calories: 320 kcal | Fat: 18 g | Protein: 28 g | Carbs: 10 g | Net carbs: 6 g | Fiber: 4 g | Cholesterol: 85 mg | Sodium: 590 mg | Potassium: 400 mg

Orange Glazed Chicken Drumsticks

Serving: 4 | Prep time: 15 minutes | Cook time: 35 minutes

Ingredients:

- 8 chicken drumsticks (about 24 oz or 680 g)
- 2 oz (60 ml) fresh orange juice
- 1 oz (30 ml) low-sodium soy sauce
- 1 oz (30 ml) honey
- 1 tsp grated orange zest
- 1 tbsp olive oil
- 2 cloves garlic, minced
- Salt and black pepper to taste
- Sesame seeds and chopped green onions for garnish

Directions:

1. Preheat your oven to 375°F (190°C).

2. In a small saucepan, combine fresh orange juice, low-sodium soy sauce, honey, and grated orange zest. Bring to a gentle boil over medium heat, then reduce the heat and simmer until the sauce thickens slightly, about 5-7 minutes. Remove from heat and set aside.

3. In a large skillet, heat olive oil over medium heat. Add minced garlic and sauté until fragrant, about 1-2 minutes.

4. Season the chicken drumsticks with salt and black pepper. Add the drumsticks to the skillet and brown them on all sides, about 3-4 minutes per side.

5. Transfer the browned drumsticks to a baking dish and brush them generously with the prepared orange glaze.

6. Bake the drumsticks in the preheated oven for 25-30 minutes or until the chicken is cooked through, and the internal temperature reaches 165°F (74°C).

Useful Tip: For an extra caramelized glaze, broil the drumsticks for 2-3 minutes after baking, watching them closely to prevent burning.

Nutritional Values: Calories: 300 kcal | Fat: 12 g | Protein: 28 g | Carbs: 20 g | Net carbs: 19 g | Fiber: 1 g | Cholesterol: 95 mg | Sodium: 350 mg | Potassium: 400 mg

Cilantro Lime Grilled Turkey Burgers

Serving: 4 | Prep time: 10 minutes | Cook time: 15 minutes

Ingredients:

- 1 lb (450 g) ground turkey
- 1 oz (30 g) fresh cilantro, chopped
- 1 oz (30 ml) lime juice
- 1 oz (30 g) red onion, finely chopped
- 1 tsp lime zest
- 2 cloves garlic, minced

- 1 tsp ground cumin
- 1/2 tsp ground coriander
- Salt and black pepper to taste
- 4 whole-grain burger buns
- Lettuce, tomato slices, and avocado slices for topping (optional)

Directions:

1. In a large mixing bowl, combine ground turkey, chopped cilantro, lime juice, finely chopped red onion, lime zest, minced garlic, ground cumin, ground coriander, salt, and black pepper. Mix well to evenly distribute the ingredients.

2. Divide the turkey mixture into 4 equal portions and shape them into burger patties.

3. Preheat your grill to medium-high heat, about 375°F to 400°F (190°C to 200°C).

4. Place the turkey patties on the preheated grill and cook for about 6-7 minutes per side or until the internal temperature reaches 165°F (74°C) and the burgers are no longer pink in the center.

5. During the last few minutes of grilling, you can toast the whole-grain burger buns on the grill until they are lightly browned.

6. Assemble your turkey burgers on the toasted buns, adding lettuce, tomato slices, and avocado slices if desired.

Useful Tip: For extra juiciness, consider brushing the burger patties with a bit of olive oil or avocado oil before grilling.

Nutritional Values: Calories: 260 kcal | Fat: 6 g | Protein: 25 g | Carbs: 27 g | Net carbs: 24 g | Fiber: 3 g | Cholesterol: 55 mg | Sodium: 370 mg | Potassium: 320 mg

Lemon Garlic Roasted Chicken Thighs

Serving: 4 | Prep time: 10 minutes | Cook time: 30 minutes

Ingredients:

- 16 oz (450 g) boneless, skinless chicken thighs
- 1 oz (30 ml) lemon juice
- 1 oz (30 g) olive oil
- 2 cloves garlic, minced
- 1 tsp lemon zest
- 1/2 tsp dried oregano
- 1/2 tsp dried thyme
- Salt and black pepper to taste
- Lemon slices for garnish (optional)
- Fresh parsley for garnish (optional)

Directions:

1. Preheat your oven to 425°F (220°C).
2. In a mixing bowl, combine lemon juice, olive oil, minced garlic, lemon zest, dried oregano, dried thyme, salt, and black pepper.
3. Place the chicken thighs in a separate bowl and pour the lemon garlic mixture over them. Ensure the chicken thighs are well coated, then let them marinate for about 10 minutes.
4. Line a baking sheet with parchment paper for easy cleanup.
5. Arrange the marinated chicken thighs on the prepared baking sheet in a single layer.
6. Roast the chicken thighs in the preheated oven for approximately 25-30 minutes or until they reach an internal temperature of 165°F (74°C) and the skin becomes crispy.
7. Garnish with lemon slices and fresh parsley, if desired.

Useful Tip: To keep the chicken moist, you can cover it with foil during the first 15 minutes of roasting and then uncover it for the remaining time to crisp up the skin.

Nutritional Values: Calories: 220 kcal | Fat: 12 g | Protein: 24 g | Carbs: 2 g | Net carbs: 1 g | Fiber: 1 g | Cholesterol: 95 mg | Sodium: 260 mg | Potassium: 280 mg

Honey Mustard Glazed Turkey Breast

Serving: 4 | Prep time: 10 minutes | Cook time: 30 minutes

Ingredients:

- 16 oz (450 g) boneless, skinless turkey breast
- 2 oz (60 ml) honey
- 1 oz (30 ml) Dijon mustard
- 1 oz (30 ml) olive oil
- 1 clove garlic, minced
- 1/2 tsp dried thyme
- Salt and black pepper to taste
- Fresh thyme sprigs for garnish (optional)

Directions:

1. Preheat your oven to 375°F (190°C).
2. In a small bowl, whisk together honey, Dijon mustard, olive oil, minced garlic, dried thyme, salt, and black pepper.
3. Place the turkey breast in a baking dish lined with foil or parchment paper for easy cleanup.
4. Pour the honey mustard mixture over the turkey breast, ensuring it's evenly coated.
5. Bake the turkey breast in the preheated oven for approximately 25-30 minutes or until it reaches an internal temperature of 165°F (74°C). Baste the turkey with the glaze halfway through the cooking time.
6. Once cooked, let the turkey breast rest for a few minutes before slicing.
7. Garnish with fresh thyme sprigs, if desired.

Useful Tip: If you want a crispier skin, you can broil the turkey breast for a few minutes after roasting, but be sure to keep a close eye on it to prevent burning.

Nutritional Values: Calories: 250 kcal | Fat: 8 g | Protein: 28 g | Carbs: 16 g | Net carbs: 15 g | Fiber: 1 g | Cholesterol: 70 mg | Sodium: 350 mg | Potassium: 310 mg

Stuffed Zucchini with Ground Chicken

Serving: 4 | Prep time: 20 minutes | Cook time: 30 minutes

Ingredients:

- 4 medium-sized zucchini (about 16 oz or 450 g each)
- 16 oz (450 g) ground chicken
- 1 small onion, finely chopped
- 2 cloves garlic, minced
- 1/2 red bell pepper, diced
- 1/2 yellow bell pepper, diced
- 2 oz (60 ml) tomato sauce
- 1 tsp dried basil
- 1 tsp dried oregano
- Salt and black pepper to taste
- 1 oz (30 g) shredded mozzarella cheese
- Fresh basil leaves for garnish (optional)

Directions:

1. Preheat your oven to 375°F (190°C).
2. Cut the tops off the zucchinis and slice them in half lengthwise. Scoop out the centers using a spoon, leaving a shell of about 1/4 inch (0.6 cm). Reserve the scooped-out flesh.
3. In a large skillet over medium heat, cook the ground chicken until it's no longer pink. Remove it from the skillet and set it aside.
4. In the same skillet, add a bit of olive oil if needed, and sauté the chopped onion, minced garlic, and diced bell peppers until they're tender.
5. Chop the reserved zucchini flesh and add it to the skillet. Cook for a few minutes until it's soft.
6. Stir in the cooked ground chicken, tomato sauce, dried basil, dried oregano, salt, and black pepper. Cook for an additional 5 minutes, allowing the flavors to meld.
7. Fill each hollowed-out zucchini with the chicken mixture and place them in a baking dish.
8. Sprinkle the shredded mozzarella cheese evenly over the stuffed zucchinis.
9. Cover the baking dish with foil and bake for 20-25 minutes, or until the zucchinis are tender.
10. If you prefer a golden, bubbly cheese topping, remove the foil and broil for a couple of minutes.
11. Garnish with fresh basil leaves, if desired.

Useful Tip: If your zucchinis are a bit watery, you can salt them lightly and let them sit for 10-15 minutes before filling to help remove excess moisture.

Nutritional Values: Calories: 290 kcal | Fat: 12 g | Protein: 27 g | Carbs: 20 g | Net carbs: 16 g | Fiber: 4 g | Cholesterol: 80 mg | Sodium: 420 mg | Potassium: 1200 mg

Baked Garlic Herb Turkey Meatballs

Serving: 4 | Prep time: 15 minutes | Cook time: 20 minutes

Ingredients:

- 16 oz (450 g) ground turkey
- 1 oz (30 g) breadcrumbs
- 1 oz (30 g) grated Parmesan cheese
- 2 oz (60 ml) unsweetened almond milk
- 2 cloves garlic, minced
- 1/2 tsp dried basil
- 1/2 tsp dried oregano
- 1/4 tsp dried thyme
- Salt and black pepper to taste
- Cooking spray (olive oil or coconut oil)
- Fresh parsley for garnish (optional)

Directions:

1. Preheat your oven to 375°F (190°C) and line a baking sheet with parchment paper or lightly grease it with cooking spray.
2. In a mixing bowl, combine the ground turkey, breadcrumbs, grated Parmesan cheese, unsweetened almond milk, minced garlic, dried basil, dried oregano, dried thyme, salt, and black pepper. Mix until all the

ingredients are well combined.

3. Using clean hands, shape the mixture into meatballs, about 1.5 inches (3.8 cm) in diameter, and place them on the prepared baking sheet.

4. Lightly spray the meatballs with cooking spray to help them brown nicely in the oven.

5. Bake the meatballs for about 20 minutes or until they are cooked through and have reached an internal temperature of 165°F (74°C).

6. If you'd like to give them a golden finish, broil for an additional 2-3 minutes.

7. Garnish with fresh parsley, if desired.

Useful Tip: For a burst of flavor, you can also add finely chopped fresh herbs like parsley or cilantro to the meatball mixture before shaping them.

Nutritional Values: Calories: 200 kcal | Fat: 9 g | Protein: 24 g | Carbs: 7 g | Net carbs: 5 g | Fiber: 2 g | Cholesterol: 70 mg | Sodium: 300 mg | Potassium: 220 mg

Rosemary and Garlic Roasted Beef Tenderloin

Serving: 4 | Prep time: 15 minutes | Cook time: 35 minutes

Ingredients:

- 1 lb (450 g) beef tenderloin
- 1 oz (28 g) fresh rosemary leaves, chopped
- 4 cloves garlic, minced
- 2 tbsp olive oil
- Salt and black pepper to taste
- Cooking spray (olive oil or coconut oil)

Directions:

1. Preheat your oven to 425°F (220°C).

2. In a small bowl, combine the chopped rosemary, minced garlic, olive oil, salt, and black pepper to create a fragrant herb mixture.

3. Place the beef tenderloin on a clean surface and rub the herb mixture evenly over the entire surface of the meat, ensuring it's well coated.

4. Heat a skillet or oven-safe pan over medium-high heat and lightly grease it with cooking spray.

5. Once the pan is hot, sear the beef tenderloin on all sides until it's nicely browned, about 2-3 minutes per side.

6. Transfer the seared beef tenderloin to a baking dish or continue roasting if your pan is oven-safe.

7. Roast the beef in the preheated oven for approximately 25-30 minutes, or until it reaches your desired level of doneness. For medium-rare, aim for an internal temperature of 135°F (57°C).

8. Remove the beef from the oven and let it rest for about 10 minutes before slicing.

Useful Tip: To ensure even cooking, it's best to let the beef come to room temperature for about 30 minutes before roasting.

Nutritional Values: Calories: 250 kcal | Fat: 16 g | Protein: 24 g | Carbs: 2 g | Net carbs: 1 g | Fiber: 1 g | Cholesterol: 75 mg | Sodium: 70 mg | Potassium: 400 mg

Grilled Herb-Marinated Quail

Serving: 4 | Prep time: 20 minutes | Cook time: 15 minutes

Ingredients:

- 4 quail (12 oz each), gutted and cleaned
- 2 oz (56 g) fresh herbs (rosemary, thyme, and oregano), finely chopped
- 4 cloves garlic, minced
- 2 oz (60 ml) olive oil
- Juice of 1 lemon
- Salt and black pepper to taste
- Cooking spray (olive oil or coconut oil)

Directions:

1. In a bowl, combine the chopped fresh herbs, minced garlic, olive oil, lemon juice, salt, and black pepper to create a flavorful herb marinade.

2. Place the quail in a large, resealable plastic bag or a shallow dish and pour the herb marinade over them. Seal the bag or cover the dish and refrigerate for at least 2 hours, allowing the quail to marinate.

3. Preheat your grill to medium-high heat, about 350-400°F (175-200°C).

4. Remove the quail from the marinade and let any excess marinade drip off. Season the quail with additional salt and pepper if desired.

5. Lightly grease the grill grates with cooking spray to prevent sticking.

6. Place the quail on the grill and cook for approximately 5-7 minutes per side, or until they reach an internal temperature of 165°F (74°C) and the skin is nicely charred and crispy.

7. Remove the grilled quail from the heat and let them rest for a few minutes before serving.

Useful Tip: To add a smoky flavor, consider using wood chips (such as apple or hickory) on your grill while cooking the quail.

Nutritional Values: Calories: 350 kcal | Fat: 24 g | Protein: 30 g | Carbs: 1 g | Net carbs: 0 g | Fiber: 0 g | Cholesterol: 140 mg | Sodium: 90 mg | Potassium: 330 mg

Braised Rabbit with Tomato and Herbs

Serving: 4 | Prep time: 20 minutes | Cook time: 2 hours

Ingredients:

- 2 lbs (900 g) rabbit, cut into serving pieces
- 4 oz (115 g) pancetta, diced
- 1 onion, finely chopped
- 2 cloves garlic, minced
- 14 oz (400 g) canned crushed tomatoes
- 8 oz (240 ml) chicken broth
- 1 sprig fresh rosemary
- 1 sprig fresh thyme
- 2 bay leaves
- Salt and black pepper to taste
- 2 tbsp olive oil
- Chopped fresh parsley for garnish

Directions:

1. Heat the olive oil in a large, heavy-bottomed pot over medium-high heat. Add the diced pancetta and cook until it becomes crispy, about 3-4 minutes. Remove the pancetta and set it aside.

2. In the same pot, add the rabbit pieces and brown them on all sides, about 5-7 minutes. Remove the rabbit and set it aside.

3. In the same pot, add the chopped onion and cook until it becomes translucent, about 3 minutes. Add the minced garlic and cook for an additional 1 minute.

4. Return the rabbit and crispy pancetta to the pot. Add the crushed tomatoes, chicken broth, rosemary, thyme, bay leaves, salt, and black pepper. Stir well to combine.

5. Bring the mixture to a simmer, then reduce the heat to low, cover, and let it gently simmer for about 1.5 to 2 hours or until the rabbit is tender and the sauce has thickened. Stir occasionally.

6. Remove the rosemary and thyme sprigs and bay leaves. Taste and adjust the seasoning, if needed.

7. Serve the braised rabbit with tomato and herbs hot, garnished with chopped fresh parsley.

Useful Tip: Rabbit can be a lean meat, but it tends to be tough, so the slow braising method in this recipe ensures it becomes tender and flavorful.

Nutritional Values: Calories: 320 kcal | Fat: 15 g | Protein: 34 g | Carbs: 12 g | Net carbs: 8 g | Fiber: 4 g | Cholesterol: 100 mg | Sodium: 760 mg | Potassium: 850 mg

Grilled Rabbit Skewers with Lemon and Garlic

Serving: 4 | Prep time: 30 minutes | Cook time: 10 minutes

Ingredients:

- 1.5 lbs (680 g) rabbit meat, cut into 1-inch (2.5 cm) pieces
- Zest and juice of 1 lemon
- 3 cloves garlic, minced
- 2 tbsp olive oil
- 1 tsp dried oregano
- Salt and black pepper to taste
- 4 metal or wooden skewers, soaked in water if wooden

Directions:

1. In a bowl, combine the lemon zest, lemon juice, minced garlic, olive oil, dried oregano, salt, and black pepper to create the marinade.
2. Place the rabbit pieces in a shallow dish or resealable plastic bag and pour the marinade over them. Ensure all the rabbit pieces are well-coated. Marinate in the refrigerator for at least 20 minutes.
3. Preheat your grill to medium-high heat (around 375°F or 190°C).
4. Thread the marinated rabbit pieces onto the skewers, leaving a small space between each piece.
5. Place the rabbit skewers on the preheated grill and cook for about 5 minutes on each side, or until they are cooked through and have grill marks. The internal temperature should reach 160°F (71°C).
6. Remove the skewers from the grill and let them rest for a few minutes.
7. Serve the grilled rabbit skewers with a fresh salad or your favorite side dishes.

Useful Tip: Rabbit meat is lean and can dry out quickly, so be careful not to overcook it. Grill until just cooked through to keep it tender and flavorful.

Nutritional Values: Calories: 220 kcal | Fat: 7 g | Protein: 36 g | Carbs: 2 g | Net carbs: 1 g | Fiber: 1 g | Cholesterol: 110 mg | Sodium: 60 mg | Potassium: 470 mg

Baked Quail with Apricot Glaze

Serving: 4 | Prep time: 20 minutes | Cook time: 25 minutes

Ingredients:

- 4 quails, cleaned and patted dry (about 16 oz or 450 g each)
- Salt and black pepper, to taste
- 2 oz (60 ml) apricot preserves
- 1 oz (30 ml) balsamic vinegar
- 1 tbsp olive oil
- 2 cloves garlic, minced
- Fresh parsley, chopped, for garnish

Directions:

1. Preheat the oven to 375°F (190°C).
2. Season the quails inside and out with salt and black pepper. Place them in a baking dish.
3. In a small saucepan, combine apricot preserves, balsamic vinegar, olive oil, and minced garlic. Heat over low heat, stirring continuously until the preserves are melted and the glaze is well combined. Remove from heat.
4. Brush the quails generously with the apricot glaze, ensuring they are well coated on all sides.
5. Bake in the preheated oven for 20-25 minutes or until the quails are cooked through, basting with the apricot glaze every 10 minutes.
6. Remove from the oven and let the quails rest for a few minutes before serving.

Useful Tip: To intensify the flavor, marinate the quails in the apricot glaze for 1-2 hours in the refrigerator before baking.

Nutritional Values: Calories: 300 kcal | Fat: 12 g | Protein: 30 g | Carbs: 15 g | Net carbs: 14 g | Fiber: 1 g | Cholesterol: 150 mg | Sodium: 80 mg | Potassium: 350 mg

Braised Veal with Tomato and Herbs

Serving: 4 | Prep time: 15 minutes | Cook time: 2 hours

Ingredients:

- 24 oz (680 g) veal stew meat, cubed
- Salt and black pepper, to taste
- 2 oz (60 ml) olive oil
- 1 onion, finely chopped
- 2 cloves garlic, minced
- 14 oz (400 g) canned diced tomatoes
- 1 tsp (5 ml) dried oregano
- 1 tsp (5 ml) dried basil
- 1 bay leaf
- Fresh parsley, chopped, for garnish

Directions:

1. Season the veal cubes with salt and black pepper.
2. In a large skillet, heat the olive oil over medium-high heat. Add the veal and sear on all sides until browned. Remove the veal from the skillet and set it aside.
3. In the same skillet, add chopped onion and minced garlic. Sauté until the onion becomes translucent.
4. Return the seared veal to the skillet and add canned diced tomatoes, dried oregano, dried basil, and a bay leaf. Stir to combine.
5. Reduce the heat to low, cover the skillet, and let it simmer for 2 hours, stirring occasionally, until the veal is tender and the sauce has thickened.
6. Remove the bay leaf before serving. Garnish with chopped fresh parsley.

Useful Tip: You can serve this braised veal with steamed vegetables or over a bed of cooked quinoa for a complete meal.

Nutritional Values: Calories: 320 kcal | Fat: 15 g | Protein: 25 g | Carbs: 16 g | Net carbs: 12 g | Fiber: 4 g | Cholesterol: 75 mg | Sodium: 480 mg | Potassium: 750 mg

Quail Stuffed with Quinoa and Vegetables

Serving: 4 | Prep time: 20 minutes | Cook time: 30 minutes

Ingredients:

- 4 quails, deboned
- 4 oz (115 g) quinoa, cooked
- 2 oz (60 ml) olive oil
- 1 small onion, finely chopped
- 2 cloves garlic, minced
- 4 oz (115 g) zucchini, diced
- 4 oz (115 g) red bell pepper, diced
- 4 oz (115 g) mushrooms, chopped
- Salt and black pepper, to taste
- 1 tsp dried thyme
- 1 tsp dried rosemary
- 4 oz (120 ml) low-sodium chicken broth
- Fresh parsley, chopped, for garnish

Directions:

1. Preheat your oven to 350°F (175°C).
2. In a large skillet, heat 2 tablespoons of olive oil over medium heat. Add chopped onion and minced garlic, and sauté until they become fragrant and translucent.
3. Add the diced zucchini, red bell pepper, and mushrooms to the skillet. Season with salt, black pepper, dried thyme, and dried rosemary. Sauté the vegetables until they are tender, about 5-7 minutes.
4. In a separate pan, heat the remaining olive oil over medium-high heat. Add the deboned quails and sear them on all sides until golden brown. Remove from heat and set aside.
5. In a bowl, combine the cooked quinoa with the sautéed vegetables. Mix well.
6. Stuff each quail with the quinoa and vegetable mixture.
7. Place the stuffed quails in a baking dish and pour the low-sodium chicken broth over them.

8. Cover the baking dish with aluminum foil and bake in the preheated oven for about 30 minutes or until the quails are cooked through.

9. Garnish with chopped fresh parsley before serving.

Useful Tip: You can serve the stuffed quails with a side of steamed asparagus or green beans for a balanced meal.

Nutritional Values: Calories: 350 kcal | Fat: 15 g | Protein: 20 g | Carbs: 30 g | Net carbs: 25 g | Fiber: 5 g | Cholesterol: 80 mg | Sodium: 280 mg | Potassium: 400 mg

Quail and Mushroom Skewers

Serving: 4 | Prep time: 20 minutes | Cook time: 15 minutes

Ingredients:

- 16 quail breasts, boneless
- 8 oz (225 g) mushrooms, cleaned and halved
- 2 oz (60 ml) olive oil
- 2 cloves garlic, minced
- 1 lemon, zested and juiced
- 1 tsp dried oregano
- Salt and black pepper, to taste
- Wooden skewers, soaked in water for 30 minutes

Directions:

1. In a bowl, combine olive oil, minced garlic, lemon zest, lemon juice, dried oregano, salt, and black pepper. Mix well to create the marinade.

2. Cut each quail breast in half, creating 32 pieces in total.

3. Place the quail pieces in the marinade, ensuring they are well coated. Allow them to marinate for at least 10 minutes, or you can refrigerate them for a few hours for more flavor.

4. Preheat your grill to medium-high heat.

5. Thread the marinated quail pieces and mushroom halves onto the soaked wooden skewers, alternating between quail and mushrooms.

6. Grill the skewers for about 7-8 minutes per side or until the quail is cooked through and has a nice char.

7. Serve the quail and mushroom skewers hot, garnished with a sprinkle of fresh lemon zest and a drizzle of the remaining marinade.

Useful Tip: These skewers are delicious when served with a side of quinoa salad and a yogurt-based tzatziki sauce.

Nutritional Values: Calories: 300 kcal | Fat: 18 g | Protein: 25 g | Carbs: 7 g | Net carbs: 5 g | Fiber: 2 g | Cholesterol: 85 mg | Sodium: 100 mg | Potassium: 520 mg

Veal Medallions in Lemon Caper Sauce

Serving: 4 | Prep time: 15 minutes | Cook time: 15 minutes

Ingredients:

- 16 veal medallions, about 4 oz (115 g) each
- 2 oz (60 ml) olive oil
- 2 cloves garlic, minced
- 1 lemon, zested and juiced
- 2 tbsp capers
- 4 oz (120 ml) chicken broth
- Salt and black pepper, to taste
- 2 tbsp unsalted butter
- Fresh parsley, chopped, for garnish

Directions:

1. Season the veal medallions with salt and black pepper on both sides.

2. In a large skillet, heat the olive oil over medium-high heat. Add the veal medallions and cook for about 2-3 minutes per side until they are nicely browned. Remove the veal from the skillet and set it aside.

3. In the same skillet, add minced garlic and cook for about 1 minute until fragrant.

4. Add the lemon zest, lemon juice, capers, and chicken broth to the skillet. Stir well and let it simmer for 2-3 minutes, allowing the sauce to reduce slightly.

5. Return the veal medallions to the skillet and cook for an additional 2-3 minutes, ensuring they are heated through.

6. Remove the skillet from the heat and stir in unsalted butter until the sauce is smooth and glossy.

7. Serve the veal medallions hot, drizzled with the lemon caper sauce and garnished with chopped fresh parsley.

Useful Tip: This dish pairs wonderfully with steamed asparagus or a simple arugula salad for a light and refreshing meal.

Nutritional Values: Calories: 300 kcal | Fat: 15 g | Protein: 30 g | Carbs: 5 g | Net carbs: 4 g | Fiber: 1 g | Cholesterol: 85 mg | Sodium: 450 mg | Potassium: 380 mg

Braised Beef with Tomatoes and Herbs

Serving: 4 | Prep time: 15 minutes | Cook time: 2 hours

Ingredients:

- 24 oz (680 g) beef chuck, cut into chunks
- 2 oz (60 ml) olive oil
- 1 onion, finely chopped
- 3 cloves garlic, minced
- 14 oz (400 g) canned diced tomatoes
- 1 tbsp tomato paste
- 8 oz (240 ml) beef broth
- 1 tsp dried basil
- 1 tsp dried oregano
- Salt and black pepper, to taste
- Fresh parsley, chopped, for garnish

Directions:

1. Heat olive oil in a large pot over medium-high heat. Add the beef chunks and brown them on all sides. Remove the beef from the pot and set it aside.

2. In the same pot, add chopped onions and cook until translucent. Add minced garlic and sauté for another minute.

3. Stir in the diced tomatoes and tomato paste. Cook for 5 minutes, allowing the tomatoes to break down and the flavors to meld.

4. Return the browned beef to the pot. Pour in the beef broth, dried basil, dried oregano, salt, and black pepper. Stir well to combine all the ingredients.

5. Cover the pot and reduce the heat to low. Let the beef simmer for 1.5 to 2 hours, or until it becomes tender and flavorful, stirring occasionally.

6. Adjust seasoning with salt and pepper if necessary. Garnish with chopped fresh parsley before serving.

Useful Tip: For a thicker sauce, you can remove some of the liquid after cooking and simmer the sauce uncovered for a few more minutes until it reaches your desired consistency.

Nutritional Values: Calories: 400 kcal | Fat: 25 g | Protein: 35 g | Carbs: 10 g | Net carbs: 7 g | Fiber: 3 g | Cholesterol: 110 mg | Sodium: 600 mg | Potassium: 900 mg

VEGETARIAN RECIPES

Spinach and Quinoa Stuffed Bell Peppers

Serving: 4 | Prep time: 20 minutes | Cook time: 45 minutes

Ingredients:

- 4 bell peppers, any color
- 6 oz (170 g) fresh spinach, chopped
- 7 oz (200 g) cooked quinoa
- 8 oz (240 ml) vegetable broth
- 1 onion, finely chopped
- 2 cloves garlic, minced
- 14 oz (400 g) canned diced tomatoes
- 2 tbsp olive oil
- 1 tsp dried oregano
- 1 tsp dried basil
- Salt and black pepper, to taste

Directions:

1. Preheat your oven to 375°F (190°C).
2. Cut the tops off the bell peppers and remove the seeds and membranes. Rinse them under cold water and set aside.
3. In a large skillet, heat olive oil over medium heat. Add chopped onions and garlic, sauté until softened.
4. Add chopped spinach to the skillet and cook until wilted.
5. Stir in cooked quinoa, diced tomatoes (with their juices), vegetable broth, dried oregano, dried basil, salt, and black pepper. Cook for a few more minutes until everything is well combined.
6. Stuff the bell peppers with the spinach and quinoa mixture, packing it tightly.
7. Place the stuffed bell peppers in a baking dish, standing upright. You can cover the dish with foil if you prefer a softer texture for the peppers.
8. Bake in the preheated oven for 30-40 minutes, or until the bell peppers are tender.
9. Serve hot.

Useful Tip: If the tops of the bell peppers start to brown too quickly, you can tent them with foil during baking.

Nutritional Values: Calories: 260 kcal | Fat: 8 g | Protein: 9 g | Carbs: 41 g | Net carbs: 31 g | Fiber: 10 g | Cholesterol: 0 mg | Sodium: 600 mg | Potassium: 800 mg

Sweet Potato and Lentil Curry

Serving: 4 | Prep time: 15 minutes | Cook time: 30 minutes

Ingredients:

- 10 oz (280 g) sweet potatoes, peeled and diced
- 6 oz (170 g) red lentils
- 1 onion, finely chopped
- 2 cloves garlic, minced
- 1-inch piece of fresh ginger, grated
- 14 oz (400 g) canned diced tomatoes
- 14 oz (400 ml) canned coconut milk
- 1 tbsp vegetable oil
- 2 tsp curry powder
- 1 tsp ground cumin
- 1 tsp ground coriander
- 1/2 tsp turmeric
- Salt and black pepper, to taste
- Fresh cilantro leaves, for garnish
- Cooked rice, for serving

Directions:

1. Heat vegetable oil in a large skillet over medium heat. Add chopped onions and sauté until they turn translucent.
2. Add minced garlic and grated ginger to the skillet, and cook for another minute until fragrant.

3. Stir in the curry powder, ground cumin, ground coriander, and turmeric. Cook for a couple of minutes to toast the spices.

4. Add the diced sweet potatoes and red lentils to the skillet, stirring to coat them with the spice mixture.

5. Pour in the canned diced tomatoes and coconut milk. Season with salt and black pepper.

6. Bring the mixture to a boil, then reduce the heat and simmer for about 20-25 minutes, or until the sweet potatoes and lentils are tender and the sauce thickens.

7. Serve the sweet potato and lentil curry over cooked rice, garnished with fresh cilantro leaves.

Useful Tip: Adjust the amount of red lentils and cooking time to achieve your desired curry consistency. For a thicker curry, use fewer lentils and simmer a bit longer; for a thinner consistency, use more lentils and reduce the simmering time.

Nutritional Values: Calories: 350 kcal | Fat: 14 g | Protein: 12 g | Carbs: 48 g | Net carbs: 34 g | Fiber: 14 g | Cholesterol: 0 mg | Sodium: 680 mg | Potassium: 860 mg

Zucchini Noodles with Pesto

Serving: 4 | Prep time: 15 minutes | Cook time: 10 minutes

Ingredients:

- 16 oz (450g) zucchini noodles
- 2 oz (60g) fresh basil leaves
- 2 oz (60g) pine nuts
- 2 oz (60g) grated Parmesan cheese
- 2 cloves garlic
- 4 oz (120ml) extra virgin olive oil
- Salt and pepper to taste
- 1 oz (30g) sun-dried tomatoes, chopped
- 2 oz (60g) black olives, sliced
- 1 oz (30g) grated Pecorino Romano cheese for garnish

Directions:

1. In a food processor, combine the fresh basil, pine nuts, grated Parmesan, and garlic. Pulse until finely chopped.

2. While the processor is running, slowly drizzle in the olive oil until the pesto reaches a smooth consistency. Season with salt and pepper to taste.

3. Heat a large skillet over medium-high heat. Add the zucchini noodles and cook for about 2-3 minutes until they are just tender, stirring occasionally. Drain any excess liquid.

4. In the same skillet, add the sun-dried tomatoes and black olives. Cook for another 2 minutes, allowing the flavors to meld.

5. Toss the cooked zucchini noodles with the freshly made pesto sauce, ensuring they are well coated.

6. Serve the zucchini noodles in individual plates, garnished with grated Pecorino Romano cheese.

7. Enjoy the dish.

Useful Tip: To make this dish even more nutritious, consider adding some roasted cherry tomatoes or grilled vegetables for extra flavor and texture.

Nutritional Values: Calories: 318 kcal | Fat: 30g | Protein: 7g | Carbs: 6g | Net carbs: 4g | Fiber: 2g | Cholesterol: 5mg | Sodium: 295mg | Potassium: 330mg

Начало формы

Creamy Mushroom Risotto

Serving: 4 | Prep time: 10 minutes | Cook time: 30 minutes

Ingredients:

- 8 oz (225g) Arborio rice
- 16 oz (450g) mixed mushrooms (such as cremini, shiitake, and oyster), sliced
- 1 oz (30g) dried porcini mushrooms
- 2 oz (60g) grated Parmesan cheese
- 2 oz (60g) butter

- 1 small onion, finely chopped
- 2 cloves garlic, minced
- 32 oz (950ml) vegetable broth, hot
- 2 tbsp olive oil
- Salt and pepper to taste
- Fresh parsley, chopped, for garnish

Directions:

1. In a heatproof bowl, soak the dried porcini mushrooms in 8 oz (240ml) of hot water for 15 minutes. Drain and reserve the soaking liquid. Chop the rehydrated porcini mushrooms.

2. In a large skillet, heat the olive oil over medium heat. Add the chopped onion and garlic and sauté until translucent, about 3 minutes.

3. Add the Arborio rice to the skillet and toast it for 2 minutes, stirring frequently until it's lightly golden.

4. Begin adding the hot vegetable broth, one ladleful at a time, stirring frequently and allowing the liquid to be absorbed before adding more. Continue this process until the rice is creamy and cooked to your desired consistency (about 18-20 minutes).

5. While cooking the risotto, in a separate pan, sauté the mixed mushrooms (including the rehydrated porcini mushrooms) in butter until they are tender and browned. Season with salt and pepper.

6. Once the risotto is creamy and the rice is cooked, stir in the grated Parmesan cheese and the sautéed mushrooms. If needed, you can also add some of the reserved porcini soaking liquid for extra flavor.

7. Season with additional salt and pepper if required, garnish with fresh parsley, and serve hot.

Useful Tip: For added richness, you can replace some of the vegetable broth with a small amount of heavy cream or coconut milk, especially if you prefer an even creamier texture.

Nutritional Values: Calories: 372 kcal | Fat: 14g | Protein: 9g | Carbs: 51g | Net carbs: 45g | Fiber: 6g | Cholesterol: 33mg | Sodium: 832mg | Potassium: 407mg

Baked Eggplant Parmesan

Serving: 4 | Prep time: 20 minutes | Cook time: 35 minutes

Ingredients:

- 2 large eggplants (about 24 oz or 680g each), sliced into 1/2-inch rounds
- 8 oz (225g) mozzarella cheese, shredded
- 4 oz (120g) grated Parmesan cheese
- 16 oz (450g) marinara sauce
- 2 oz (60g) breadcrumbs
- 2 oz (60g) almond flour
- 2 eggs
- 1 tsp olive oil
- 1 tsp Italian seasoning
- Salt and pepper to taste
- Fresh basil leaves for garnish

Directions:

1. Preheat your oven to 375°F (190°C).

2. In a shallow bowl, whisk the eggs with a teaspoon of olive oil and a pinch of salt and pepper.

3. In a separate bowl, combine the breadcrumbs, almond flour, Italian seasoning, and half of the grated Parmesan cheese.

4. Dip each eggplant slice into the egg mixture, ensuring it's well coated, then coat it with the breadcrumb mixture.

5. Place the coated eggplant slices on a baking sheet lined with parchment paper and bake for 15-20 minutes, flipping them halfway through, until they are golden brown.

6. In a separate baking dish, spread a thin layer of marinara sauce, then add a layer of baked eggplant slices.

7. Top the eggplant with a layer of shredded mozzarella cheese and some grated Parmesan.

8. Repeat the layers until all the ingredients are used, finishing with a layer of marinara sauce and cheese on top.

9. Bake in the preheated oven for an additional 15-20 minutes, until the cheese is bubbly and golden.

10. Garnish with fresh basil leaves before serving.

Useful Tip: For a lighter version of this dish, you can use part-skim mozzarella cheese and whole wheat breadcrumbs to reduce the fat content and increase the fiber. Enjoy the dish!

Nutritional Values: Calories: 384 kcal | Fat: 24g | Protein: 23g | Carbs: 24g | Net carbs: 18g | Fiber: 6g | Cholesterol: 119mg | Sodium: 946mg | Potassium: 667mg

Cauliflower and Broccoli Bake

Serving: 4 | Prep time: 15 minutes | Cook time: 30 minutes

Ingredients:

- 12 oz (340g) cauliflower florets
- 12 oz (340g) broccoli florets
- 4 oz (120g) shredded cheddar cheese
- 4 oz (120g) sour cream
- 2 oz (60g) cream cheese
- 2 oz (60ml) almond milk
- 1 oz (30g) grated Parmesan cheese
- 1/2 tsp garlic powder
- 1/2 tsp onion powder
- Salt and pepper to taste
- 2 oz (60g) crushed pork rinds (optional, for a crunchy topping)
- Fresh parsley for garnish

Directions:

1. Preheat your oven to 375°F (190°C).
2. Steam the cauliflower and broccoli florets until they are slightly tender, about 5 minutes. Drain and set aside.
3. In a saucepan over medium heat, combine the cream cheese, sour cream, almond milk, garlic powder, onion powder, half of the shredded cheddar cheese, and half of the grated Parmesan cheese. Stir until the cheeses are melted and the mixture is smooth.
4. Season the cheese mixture with salt and pepper to taste.
5. In a large mixing bowl, gently fold the steamed cauliflower and broccoli into the cheese sauce until they are well coated.
6. Transfer the mixture to a baking dish and sprinkle the remaining shredded cheddar cheese and grated Parmesan cheese on top.
7. If desired, sprinkle the crushed pork rinds over the cheese layer for added crunch.
8. Bake in the preheated oven for 20-25 minutes, or until the top is golden brown and bubbling.
9. Garnish with fresh parsley before serving.

Useful Tip: For a gluten-free option, skip the crushed pork rinds. This creamy and cheesy cauliflower and broccoli bake is a satisfying side dish that complements any meal. Enjoy the dish!

Nutritional Values: Calories: 305 kcal | Fat: 24g | Protein: 12g | Carbs: 11g | Net carbs: 7g | Fiber: 4g | Cholesterol: 58mg | Sodium: 467mg | Potassium: 479mg

Начало формы

Grilled Portobello Mushrooms with Balsamic Glaze

Serving: 4 | Prep time: 10 minutes | Cook time: 15 minutes

Ingredients:

- 4 large Portobello mushrooms (about 24 oz or 680g)
- 2 oz (60ml) balsamic vinegar
- 2 oz (60ml) olive oil
- 2 cloves garlic, minced
- 1 tsp dried thyme
- Salt and pepper to taste
- Fresh parsley, chopped, for garnish

Directions:

1. Preheat your grill to medium-high heat (about 400°F or 200°C).

2. In a small bowl, whisk together the balsamic vinegar, olive oil, minced garlic, dried thyme, salt, and pepper to create the marinade.

3. Clean the Portobello mushrooms by gently wiping them with a damp cloth or paper towel to remove any dirt. Remove the stems and gills.

4. Place the mushrooms in a shallow dish and pour the balsamic marinade over them. Allow them to marinate for about 5-10 minutes, turning them occasionally to coat evenly.

5. Place the marinated Portobello mushrooms on the preheated grill, cap side down.

6. Grill for about 5-7 minutes on each side, or until they are tender and have grill marks.

7. While grilling, baste the mushrooms with the remaining marinade to enhance the flavor.

8. Remove the grilled Portobello mushrooms from the grill and garnish with fresh chopped parsley.

9. Serve hot as a side dish or as a main course.

Useful Tip: For extra flavor, you can add a sprinkle of crumbled goat cheese or feta on top of the grilled Portobello mushrooms just before serving. Enjoy the dish!

Nutritional Values: Calories: 105 kcal | Fat: 9g | Protein: 2g | Carbs: 4g | Net carbs: 3g | Fiber: 1g | Cholesterol: 0mg | Sodium: 10mg | Potassium: 416mg

Ratatouille

Serving: 4 | Prep time: 20 minutes | Cook time: 40 minutes

Ingredients:

- 2 medium-sized eggplants (about 24 oz or 680g), diced
- 2 zucchinis (about 12 oz or 340g), diced
- 2 red bell peppers (about 12 oz or 340g), diced
- 2 yellow onions (about 8 oz or 225g), diced
- 4 cloves garlic, minced
- 16 oz (450g) canned diced tomatoes
- 4 oz (120ml) tomato paste
- 2 oz (60ml) olive oil
- 1 tsp dried thyme
- 1 tsp dried oregano
- Salt and pepper to taste
- Fresh basil leaves for garnish

Directions:

1. Heat the olive oil in a large skillet or Dutch oven over medium heat.

2. Add the diced onions and minced garlic. Sauté until the onions become translucent, about 3-4 minutes.

3. Add the diced eggplants, zucchinis, and red bell peppers to the skillet. Cook for about 10-12 minutes, or until they start to soften.

4. Stir in the diced tomatoes and tomato paste. Mix well.

5. Season the mixture with dried thyme, dried oregano, salt, and pepper.

6. Cover and simmer for about 20-25 minutes, stirring occasionally, until the vegetables are tender and the flavors have melded together.

7. Adjust the seasoning if needed.

8. Garnish with fresh basil leaves before serving.

Useful Tip: Ratatouille can be enjoyed hot or cold. It's a versatile dish that can be served as a side, over pasta, on top of crusty bread, or as a main course. Experiment with different herbs and spices to suit your taste preferences. Enjoy the dish!

Nutritional Values: Calories: 178 kcal | Fat: 7g | Protein: 3g | Carbs: 29g | Net carbs: 20g | Fiber: 9g | Cholesterol: 0mg | Sodium: 298mg | Potassium: 1052mg

Roasted Butternut Squash and Apple Salad

Serving: 4 | Prep time: 15 minutes | Cook time: 25 minutes

Ingredients:

- 16 oz (450g) butternut squash, peeled, seeded, and diced
- 12 oz (340g) apples (such as Granny Smith or Honeycrisp), diced
- 4 oz (120g) mixed greens (e.g., arugula, spinach, or lettuce)
- 2 oz (60g) dried cranberries
- 2 oz (60g) pecans, chopped
- 2 oz (60ml) olive oil
- 2 oz (60ml) balsamic vinegar
- 1 oz (30g) honey
- 1/2 tsp cinnamon
- Salt and pepper to taste

Directions:

1. Preheat your oven to 400°F (200°C).
2. In a large mixing bowl, combine the diced butternut squash, olive oil, cinnamon, salt, and pepper. Toss until the squash is well coated.
3. Spread the seasoned butternut squash on a baking sheet and roast for 20-25 minutes or until it's tender and lightly caramelized, stirring once or twice during cooking.
4. While the squash is roasting, prepare the dressing. In a small bowl, whisk together the balsamic vinegar and honey until well combined. Set aside.
5. Once the butternut squash is done, let it cool for a few minutes.
6. In a large salad bowl, combine the mixed greens, diced apples, dried cranberries, and chopped pecans.
7. Add the roasted butternut squash to the salad ingredients.
8. Drizzle the dressing over the salad and toss gently to combine.
9. Season with additional salt and pepper to taste.
10. Serve immediately.

Useful Tip: To make this salad more substantial, you can add crumbled feta or goat cheese for some creaminess and extra flavor. Enjoy the dish!

Nutritional Values: Calories: 323 kcal | Fat: 18g | Protein: 3g | Carbs: 43g | Net carbs: 32g | Fiber: 11g | Cholesterol: 0mg | Sodium: 16mg | Potassium: 694mg

Cucumber and Dill Greek Yogurt Dip

Serving: 4 | Prep time: 10 minutes | Cook time: 0 minutes

Ingredients:

- 16 oz (450g) Greek yogurt
- 4 oz (120g) cucumber, finely grated and excess water squeezed out
- 1 oz (30g) fresh dill, finely chopped
- 2 cloves garlic, minced
- 1 oz (30ml) lemon juice
- 1 oz (30ml) olive oil
- Salt and pepper to taste
- Fresh cucumber slices and dill sprigs for garnish

Directions:

1. In a mixing bowl, combine the Greek yogurt, finely grated cucumber, minced garlic, and chopped fresh dill.
2. Add the lemon juice and olive oil to the mixture, and stir until everything is well incorporated.
3. Season the dip with salt and pepper to taste, adjusting the seasonings as needed.
4. Refrigerate the dip for at least 30 minutes to allow the flavors to meld.
5. Before serving, garnish with fresh cucumber slices and dill sprigs.
6. Serve the cucumber and dill Greek yogurt dip with your choice of sliced vegetables or whole-grain crackers.

Useful Tip: For a creamier texture, you can add a touch of mayonnaise or sour cream, but be mindful of the fat content if you're following a low-fat diet. Enjoy the dish as a healthy and refreshing dip or a condiment for various dishes.

Nutritional Values: Calories: 118 kcal | Fat: 7g | Protein: 7g | Carbs: 6g | Net carbs: 4g | Fiber: 2g | Cholesterol: 2mg | Sodium: 32mg | Potassium: 297mg

Spinach and Feta Stuffed Tomatoes

Serving: 4 | Prep time: 15 minutes | Cook time: 20 minutes

Ingredients:

- 4 large tomatoes (about 32 oz or 900g)
- 8 oz (225g) fresh spinach, chopped
- 4 oz (120g) feta cheese, crumbled
- 2 oz (60g) red onion, finely chopped
- 2 cloves garlic, minced
- 2 oz (60ml) olive oil
- 1 oz (30g) fresh basil leaves, chopped
- 1 oz (30g) fresh parsley, chopped
- Salt and pepper to taste

Directions:

1. Preheat your oven to 375°F (190°C).
2. Cut the tops off the tomatoes and scoop out the seeds and flesh, leaving a hollow shell. Reserve the removed flesh for later use.
3. In a large skillet, heat the olive oil over medium heat. Add the minced garlic and chopped red onion. Sauté until softened, about 2-3 minutes.
4. Add the chopped spinach and reserved tomato flesh to the skillet. Cook until the spinach wilts and the mixture is well combined, about 5 minutes.
5. Remove the skillet from the heat and stir in the crumbled feta cheese, fresh basil, and fresh parsley. Season with salt and pepper to taste.
6. Stuff each hollowed-out tomato with the spinach and feta mixture, pressing it down gently.
7. Place the stuffed tomatoes in a baking dish and bake in the preheated oven for 15-20 minutes, or until the tomatoes are tender and the stuffing is heated through.
8. Garnish with additional fresh herbs before serving.

Useful Tip: You can customize the stuffing by adding some chopped olives, pine nuts, or sun-dried tomatoes for extra flavor and texture. Enjoy the dish as a flavorful and nutritious appetizer or side dish.

Nutritional Values: Calories: 180 kcal | Fat: 15g | Protein: 6g | Carbs: 7g | Net carbs: 4g | Fiber: 3g | Cholesterol: 25mg | Sodium: 334mg | Potassium: 603mg

Roasted Brussels Sprouts with Maple Dijon Glaze

Serving: 4 | Prep time: 10 minutes | Cook time: 20 minutes

Ingredients:

- 16 oz (450g) Brussels sprouts, trimmed and halved
- 2 oz (60ml) olive oil
- 1 oz (30ml) pure maple syrup
- 1 oz (30ml) Dijon mustard
- 1 oz (30ml) balsamic vinegar
- 2 oz (60g) chopped pecans
- Salt and pepper to taste
- Fresh thyme leaves for garnish

Directions:

1. Preheat your oven to 400°F (200°C).
2. In a mixing bowl, toss the halved Brussels sprouts with olive oil, salt, and pepper until they are well coated.
3. Spread the Brussels sprouts in a single layer on a baking sheet.
4. Roast in the preheated oven for 15-20 minutes, or until they are tender and have crispy edges, stirring

halfway through cooking.

5. While the Brussels sprouts are roasting, prepare the glaze. In a small saucepan, combine maple syrup, Dijon mustard, and balsamic vinegar.

6. Heat the mixture over low heat, stirring constantly until it thickens slightly, about 2-3 minutes.

7. Remove the roasted Brussels sprouts from the oven and drizzle the maple Dijon glaze over them.

8. Toss to coat the Brussels sprouts evenly with the glaze.

9. Sprinkle the chopped pecans over the Brussels sprouts and return them to the oven for an additional 3-5 minutes, or until the pecans are lightly toasted.

10. Garnish with fresh thyme leaves before serving.

Useful Tip: For an extra burst of flavor, consider adding a sprinkle of grated Parmesan cheese to the roasted Brussels sprouts just before serving. Enjoy the dish as a delicious and nutritious side!

Nutritional Values: Calories: 238 kcal | Fat: 18g | Protein: 4g | Carbs: 19g | Net carbs: 15g | Fiber: 4g | Cholesterol: 0mg | Sodium: 156mg | Potassium: 449mg

Eggplant and Chickpea Curry

Serving: 4 | Prep time: 15 minutes | Cook time: 25 minutes

Ingredients:

- 16 oz (450g) eggplant, diced
- 14 oz (400g) canned chickpeas, drained and rinsed
- 8 oz (225g) canned diced tomatoes
- 4 oz (120ml) coconut milk
- 2 oz (60g) onion, finely chopped
- 2 cloves garlic, minced
- 2 oz (60ml) vegetable broth

- 1 oz (30g) tomato paste
- 1 oz (30ml) olive oil
- 1 tsp curry powder
- 1/2 tsp ground turmeric
- 1/2 tsp ground cumin
- Salt and pepper to taste
- Fresh cilantro leaves for garnish

Directions:

1. In a large skillet, heat the olive oil over medium heat. Add the chopped onion and minced garlic, sautéing until the onion is translucent, about 3-4 minutes.

2. Add the diced eggplant to the skillet and cook until it starts to soften, about 5 minutes.

3. Stir in the curry powder, ground turmeric, and ground cumin, cooking for another 2 minutes to toast the spices.

4. Add the canned diced tomatoes, tomato paste, and vegetable broth. Stir well to combine.

5. Cover and simmer the mixture over low heat for 10 minutes, allowing the flavors to meld and the eggplant to fully cook.

6. Add the drained and rinsed chickpeas to the skillet, stirring to combine. Cook for an additional 5 minutes.

7. Pour in the coconut milk, stirring continuously until the curry is well mixed and heated through.

8. Season the curry with salt and pepper to taste.

9. Garnish with fresh cilantro leaves before serving.

Useful Tip: Enjoy the dish served over rice or with naan bread for a satisfying, flavorful meal!

Nutritional Values: Calories: 232 kcal | Fat: 12g | Protein: 7g | Carbs: 27g | Net carbs: 18g | Fiber: 9g | Cholesterol: 0mg | Sodium: 458mg | Potassium: 777mg

Sweet Potato and Black Bean Tacos

Serving: 4 | Prep time: 15 minutes | Cook time: 25 minutes

Ingredients:

- 16 oz (450g) sweet potatoes, peeled and diced
- 8 oz (225g) canned black beans, drained and rinsed
- 4 oz (120g) red onion, finely chopped
- 4 oz (120ml) vegetable broth
- 2 oz (60g) corn kernels
- 2 oz (60ml) olive oil
- 2 oz (60ml) lime juice
- 1 oz (30g) fresh cilantro, chopped
- 1 tsp ground cumin
- 1/2 tsp chili powder
- Salt and pepper to taste
- 8 small corn tortillas

Directions:

1. In a large skillet, heat the olive oil over medium heat. Add the chopped red onion and sauté until it becomes translucent, about 3-4 minutes.

2. Add the diced sweet potatoes to the skillet and cook until they begin to soften, stirring occasionally, for about 10 minutes.

3. Stir in the ground cumin and chili powder, cooking for an additional 2 minutes to toast the spices.

4. Pour in the vegetable broth, cover, and simmer for 10-12 minutes, or until the sweet potatoes are tender and the liquid is absorbed.

5. Add the drained and rinsed black beans and corn kernels to the skillet. Cook for an additional 3-4 minutes, until they are heated through.

6. Remove the skillet from heat and drizzle lime juice over the mixture. Stir in the chopped cilantro, and season with salt and pepper to taste.

7. Warm the corn tortillas according to package instructions.

8. Spoon the sweet potato and black bean mixture onto each tortilla.

9. Serve the tacos with your favorite toppings such as avocado slices, salsa, or shredded cheese.

Useful Tip: To make these tacos even more nutritious, consider adding fresh diced tomatoes or red bell peppers for extra color and flavor. Enjoy these delicious and satisfying vegetarian tacos!

Nutritional Values: Calories: 308 kcal | Fat: 10g | Protein: 7g | Carbs: 50g | Net carbs: 34g | Fiber: 9g | Cholesterol: 0mg | Sodium: 475mg | Potassium: 637mg

SOUPS

Butternut Squash Soup

Serving: 4 | Prep time: 15 minutes | Cook time: 30 minutes

Ingredients:

- 24 oz (680g) butternut squash, peeled and diced
- 8 oz (225g) carrots, peeled and sliced
- 4 oz (120g) onion, finely chopped
- 2 cloves garlic, minced
- 2 oz (60ml) olive oil
- 32 oz (960ml) vegetable broth
- 4 oz (120ml) coconut milk
- 1 oz (30ml) maple syrup
- 1/2 tsp ground ginger
- Salt and pepper to taste
- Fresh thyme leaves for garnish

Directions:

1. In a large pot, heat the olive oil over medium heat. Add the chopped onion and minced garlic, sautéing until the onion is soft and translucent, about 3-4 minutes.
2. Add the diced butternut squash and sliced carrots to the pot. Cook for another 5 minutes, stirring occasionally.
3. Pour in the vegetable broth and add the ground ginger. Bring the mixture to a boil, then reduce the heat to a simmer. Cover and cook for about 20-25 minutes, or until the vegetables are tender.
4. Remove the pot from heat and allow the soup to cool slightly.
5. Using an immersion blender or a regular blender (in batches), puree the soup until it's smooth and creamy.
6. Return the pureed soup to the pot and place it back on the stove over low heat.
7. Stir in the coconut milk and maple syrup, mixing well to combine.
8. Season with salt and pepper to taste.
9. Heat the soup for an additional 5 minutes until it's heated through.
10. Garnish with fresh thyme leaves before serving.

Useful Tip: For added richness, you can top each bowl of soup with a dollop of Greek yogurt or a sprinkle of toasted pumpkin seeds. Enjoy this comforting and nutritious soup as a warm and satisfying meal!

Nutritional Values: Calories: 203 kcal | Fat: 10g | Protein: 2g | Carbs: 30g | Net carbs: 20g | Fiber: 10g | Cholesterol: 0mg | Sodium: 913mg | Potassium: 710mg

Lentil and Vegetable Soup

Serving: 4 | Prep time: 15 minutes | Cook time: 30 minutes

Ingredients:

- 8 oz (225g) dried green lentils
- 4 oz (120g) carrots, peeled and diced
- 4 oz (120g) celery, diced
- 4 oz (120g) onion, finely chopped
- 2 cloves garlic, minced
- 2 oz (60ml) olive oil
- 64 oz (1920ml) vegetable broth
- 4 oz (120ml) tomato sauce
- 2 oz (60ml) lemon juice
- 1 tsp ground cumin
- 1/2 tsp ground coriander
- Salt and pepper to taste
- Fresh parsley leaves for garnish

Directions:

1. Rinse the dried lentils under cold water and set them aside.

2. In a large pot, heat the olive oil over medium heat. Add the chopped onion and minced garlic, sautéing until the onion is soft and translucent, about 3-4 minutes.

3. Add the diced carrots and celery to the pot, cooking for an additional 5 minutes until they begin to soften.

4. Stir in the ground cumin and ground coriander, toasting the spices for about 2 minutes.

5. Pour in the vegetable broth, tomato sauce, and dried lentils. Bring the mixture to a boil, then reduce the heat to a simmer. Cover and cook for about 20-25 minutes, or until the lentils are tender.

6. Stir in the lemon juice and season with salt and pepper to taste.

7. Let the soup simmer for an additional 5 minutes.

8. Garnish with fresh parsley leaves before serving.

Useful Tip: To add extra flavor and a hint of freshness, consider adding a dollop of Greek yogurt or a squeeze of fresh lemon juice to each bowl of soup just before serving. Enjoy this hearty and nutritious lentil and vegetable soup!

Nutritional Values: Calories: 295 kcal | Fat: 8g | Protein: 13g | Carbs: 45g | Net carbs: 32g | Fiber: 13g | Cholesterol: 0mg | Sodium: 1353mg | Potassium: 832mg

Creamy Potato Leek Soup

Serving: 4 | Prep time: 15 minutes | Cook time: 30 minutes

Ingredients:

- 16 oz (450g) potatoes, peeled and diced
- 8 oz (225g) leeks, white and light green parts, sliced
- 4 oz (120g) onion, finely chopped
- 2 cloves garlic, minced
- 2 oz (60ml) olive oil
- 32 oz (960ml) vegetable broth
- 4 oz (120ml) milk
- 2 oz (60ml) heavy cream
- 2 oz (60g) unsalted butter
- Salt and pepper to taste
- Fresh chives for garnish

Directions:

1. In a large pot, heat the olive oil over medium heat. Add the chopped onion and minced garlic, sautéing until the onion is soft and translucent, about 3-4 minutes.

2. Add the sliced leeks to the pot and cook for an additional 5 minutes, until they begin to soften.

3. Stir in the diced potatoes and continue to cook for another 5 minutes.

4. Pour in the vegetable broth, cover, and simmer for about 15-20 minutes, or until the potatoes are tender.

5. Using an immersion blender or a regular blender (in batches), puree the soup until it's smooth.

6. Return the pureed soup to the pot and place it back on the stove over low heat.

7. Stir in the milk, heavy cream, and unsalted butter. Mix well to combine.

8. Season with salt and pepper to taste.

9. Heat the soup for an additional 5 minutes until it's heated through.

10. Garnish with fresh chives before serving.

Useful Tip: For an extra touch of flavor, consider adding a sprinkle of grated Parmesan cheese or a dollop of sour cream to each bowl of soup. Enjoy this creamy and comforting potato leek soup!

Nutritional Values: Calories: 308 kcal | Fat: 20g | Protein: 4g | Carbs: 30g | Net carbs: 20g | Fiber: 6g | Cholesterol: 47mg | Sodium: 960mg | Potassium: 752mg

Tomato Basil Soup

Serving: 4 | Prep time: 10 minutes | Cook time: 25 minutes

Ingredients:

- 24 oz (680g) canned crushed tomatoes
- 4 oz (120g) onion, finely chopped
- 4 oz (120g) carrots, peeled and diced
- 2 cloves garlic, minced
- 2 oz (60ml) olive oil
- 32 oz (960ml) vegetable broth
- 2 oz (60ml) heavy cream
- 1 oz (30g) fresh basil leaves, chopped
- 1/2 tsp dried oregano
- Salt and pepper to taste
- Grated Parmesan cheese for garnish (optional)

Directions:

1. In a large pot, heat the olive oil over medium heat. Add the chopped onion and minced garlic, sautéing until the onion is soft and translucent, about 3-4 minutes.
2. Add the diced carrots to the pot and cook for an additional 5 minutes, until they begin to soften.
3. Stir in the canned crushed tomatoes and dried oregano, cooking for another 5 minutes.
4. Pour in the vegetable broth, cover, and simmer for about 15 minutes.
5. Using an immersion blender or a regular blender (in batches), puree the soup until it's smooth.
6. Return the pureed soup to the pot and place it back on the stove over low heat.
7. Stir in the heavy cream and fresh basil. Mix well to combine.
8. Season with salt and pepper to taste.
9. Heat the soup for an additional 5 minutes until it's heated through.
10. Garnish with grated Parmesan cheese if desired.

Useful Tip: For added flavor, you can serve this delicious tomato basil soup with a drizzle of extra-virgin olive oil and a sprinkle of fresh basil leaves on top. Enjoy this classic comfort soup!

Nutritional Values: Calories: 236 kcal | Fat: 14g | Protein: 4g | Carbs: 26g | Net carbs: 18g | Fiber: 8g | Cholesterol: 20mg | Sodium: 948mg | Potassium: 830mg

Mushroom Barley Soup

Serving: 4 | Prep time: 10 minutes | Cook time: 35 minutes

Ingredients:

- 4 oz (115g) pearl barley
- 8 oz (225g) mushrooms, sliced
- 4 oz (120g) carrots, peeled and diced
- 4 oz (120g) celery, diced
- 4 oz (120g) onion, finely chopped
- 2 cloves garlic, minced
- 2 oz (60ml) olive oil
- 32 oz (960ml) vegetable broth
- 1 tsp dried thyme
- Salt and pepper to taste
- Fresh parsley leaves for garnish

Directions:

1. Rinse the pearl barley under cold water and set it aside.
2. In a large pot, heat the olive oil over medium heat. Add the chopped onion and minced garlic, sautéing until the onion is soft and translucent, about 3-4 minutes.
3. Add the sliced mushrooms, diced carrots, and diced celery to the pot. Cook for an additional 5 minutes, until the vegetables begin to soften.
4. Stir in the rinsed pearl barley and dried thyme, toasting them for about 2 minutes.
5. Add the vegetable broth, cover, and simmer for about 20-25 minutes, or until the barley is tender.
6. Season with salt and pepper to taste.

7. Let the soup simmer for an additional 5 minutes.

8. Garnish with fresh parsley leaves before serving.

Useful Tip: For extra depth of flavor, consider adding a splash of balsamic vinegar to your bowl of mushroom barley soup just before serving. Enjoy the hearty and nutritious goodness of this soup!

Nutritional Values: Calories: 272 kcal | Fat: 9g | Protein: 5g | Carbs: 42g | Net carbs: 34g | Fiber: 8g | Cholesterol: 0mg | Sodium: 720mg | Potassium: 385mg

Minestrone Soup

Serving: 4 | Prep time: 15 minutes | Cook time: 30 minutes

Ingredients:

- 4 oz (115g) small pasta (such as ditalini or small shells)
- 4 oz (115g) zucchini, diced
- 4 oz (115g) carrots, peeled and diced
- 4 oz (115g) celery, diced
- 4 oz (115g) onion, finely chopped
- 2 cloves garlic, minced
- 4 oz (120ml) olive oil

- 32 oz (960ml) vegetable broth
- 24 oz (680g) canned diced tomatoes
- 4 oz (115g) green beans, trimmed and cut into 1-inch pieces
- 4 oz (115g) kidney beans, drained and rinsed
- 1 tsp dried basil
- Salt and pepper to taste
- Grated Parmesan cheese for garnish (optional)

Directions:

1. Cook the small pasta according to package instructions until al dente. Drain and set aside.

2. In a large pot, heat the olive oil over medium heat. Add the chopped onion and minced garlic, sautéing until the onion is soft and translucent, about 3-4 minutes.

3. Add the diced zucchini, carrots, and celery to the pot. Cook for an additional 5 minutes until the vegetables begin to soften.

4. Pour in the vegetable broth and canned diced tomatoes (with their juices). Stir to combine.

5. Add the green beans and kidney beans to the pot.

6. Season with dried basil, salt, and pepper to taste. Stir well.

7. Cover and simmer for about 20-25 minutes, or until all the vegetables are tender.

8. Stir in the cooked pasta and heat for an additional 5 minutes.

9. Serve hot, garnished with grated Parmesan cheese if desired.

Useful Tip: For a burst of freshness and added flavor, sprinkle some freshly chopped basil or parsley on top of your bowl of minestrone soup just before serving. Enjoy this hearty Italian classic!

Nutritional Values: Calories: 329 kcal | Fat: 13g | Protein: 10g | Carbs: 45g | Net carbs: 32g | Fiber: 13g | Cholesterol: 0mg | Sodium: 900mg | Potassium: 930mg

Cauliflower and Broccoli Soup

Serving: 4 | Prep time: 15 minutes | Cook time: 25 minutes

Ingredients:

- 8 oz (230g) cauliflower florets
- 8 oz (230g) broccoli florets
- 4 oz (115g) leeks, chopped
- 2 cloves garlic, minced
- 4 oz (115g) celery, chopped
- 4 oz (115g) carrots, chopped

- 4 oz (115g) onion, chopped
- 32 oz (960ml) vegetable broth
- 8 oz (230ml) unsweetened almond milk (or any plant-based milk)
- 1 tsp olive oil
- Salt and pepper to taste
- Fresh parsley for garnish (optional)

Directions:

1. In a large pot, heat the olive oil over medium heat. Add the chopped onion and minced garlic, sautéing until the onion is soft and translucent, about 3-4 minutes.

2. Add the chopped leeks, celery, and carrots to the pot. Cook for an additional 5 minutes until the vegetables begin to soften.

3. Pour in the vegetable broth and bring it to a boil.

4. Add the cauliflower and broccoli florets to the pot. Reduce the heat to a simmer and cover. Cook for about 15-20 minutes, or until the vegetables are tender.

5. Using an immersion blender or a regular blender, puree the soup until smooth. Be careful when blending hot liquids.

6. Return the pureed soup to the pot, and stir in the unsweetened almond milk.

7. Season with salt and pepper to taste. Heat the soup over low heat for an additional 5 minutes, stirring occasionally.

8. Serve hot, garnished with fresh parsley if desired.

Useful Tip: For added flavor, consider sprinkling a pinch of grated Parmesan cheese or a drizzle of olive oil on top of your bowl of cauliflower and broccoli soup just before serving. Enjoy this creamy and nutritious soup!

Nutritional Values: Calories: 105 kcal | Fat: 3g | Protein: 4g | Carbs: 17g | Net carbs: 10g | Fiber: 7g | Cholesterol: 0mg | Sodium: 810mg | Potassium: 560mg

Sweet Potato and Ginger Soup

Serving: 4 | Prep time: 15 minutes | Cook time: 25 minutes

Ingredients:

- 12 oz (340g) sweet potatoes, peeled and cubed
- 2 oz (57g) onions, chopped
- 2 oz (57g) carrots, chopped
- 2 oz (57g) celery, chopped
- 1-inch piece of fresh ginger, peeled and minced
- 32 oz (960ml) vegetable broth
- 4 oz (115ml) unsweetened coconut milk
- 1 tsp olive oil
- Salt and pepper to taste
- Fresh cilantro for garnish (optional)

Directions:

1. In a large pot, heat the olive oil over medium heat. Add the chopped onions and cook until they become translucent, about 3-4 minutes.

2. Stir in the chopped carrots, celery, and minced ginger. Sauté for an additional 3-4 minutes.

3. Add the sweet potato cubes and vegetable broth to the pot. Bring to a boil, then reduce the heat to a simmer. Cover and cook for 15-20 minutes, or until the sweet potatoes are tender.

4. Using an immersion blender or a regular blender, puree the soup until it's smooth. Be cautious when blending hot liquids.

5. Return the pureed soup to the pot, and stir in the unsweetened coconut milk.

6. Season with salt and pepper to taste. Heat the soup over low heat for an additional 5 minutes, stirring occasionally.

7. Serve hot, garnished with fresh cilantro if desired.

Useful Tip: For an extra burst of flavor, you can add a squeeze of fresh lime juice just before serving. This sweet potato and ginger soup is a delightful and nutritious choice for a gallbladder-friendly meal. Enjoy!

Nutritional Values: Calories: 150 kcal | Fat: 5g | Protein: 2g | Carbs: 24g | Net carbs: 15g | Fiber: 9g | Cholesterol: 0mg | Sodium: 780mg | Potassium: 450mg

Spinach and Rice Soup

Serving: 4 | Prep time: 10 minutes | Cook time: 25 minutes

Ingredients:

- 4 oz (115g) fresh spinach, chopped
- 2 oz (57g) white rice
- 2 oz (57g) onions, finely chopped
- 2 oz (57g) carrots, diced
- 2 oz (57g) celery, diced
- 32 oz (960ml) vegetable broth
- 2 oz (57g) unsalted butter
- 2 oz (57ml) heavy cream
- 1 tsp olive oil
- Salt and pepper to taste
- Fresh parsley for garnish (optional)

Directions:

1. In a large pot, heat the olive oil and melt the butter over medium heat. Add the chopped onions, carrots, and celery. Sauté until they start to soften, about 3-4 minutes.
2. Stir in the white rice and continue to sauté for an additional 2 minutes.
3. Pour in the vegetable broth and bring the mixture to a boil. Reduce the heat to a simmer, cover, and cook for 15-20 minutes, or until the rice is tender.
4. Add the chopped spinach to the pot and simmer for an additional 5 minutes until the spinach wilts.
5. Stir in the heavy cream and season the soup with salt and pepper to taste. Cook for an additional 2-3 minutes.
6. Serve hot, garnished with fresh parsley if desired.

Useful Tip: To make this soup even heartier, consider adding some diced cooked chicken or tofu for extra protein. This Spinach and Rice Soup is a comforting and nutritious option for those on a gallbladder diet. Enjoy!

Nutritional Values: Calories: 250 kcal | Fat: 16g | Protein: 3g | Carbs: 24g | Net carbs: 20g | Fiber: 4g | Cholesterol: 50mg | Sodium: 780mg | Potassium: 370mg

Vegan Split Pea Soup

Serving: 4 | Prep time: 10 minutes | Cook time: 45 minutes

Ingredients:

- 8 oz (227g) split green peas
- 2 oz (57g) carrots, diced
- 2 oz (57g) celery, diced
- 2 oz (57g) onions, diced
- 2 cloves garlic, minced
- 2 oz (57g) potatoes, diced
- 2 oz (57g) leeks, chopped
- 1 bay leaf
- 32 oz (960ml) vegetable broth
- 16 oz (480ml) water
- 1 tsp olive oil
- Salt and pepper to taste
- Fresh parsley for garnish (optional)

Directions:

1. Rinse the split peas under cold water and set them aside.
2. In a large pot, heat the olive oil over medium heat. Add the onions, garlic, leeks, carrots, and celery. Sauté until the vegetables start to soften, about 5 minutes.
3. Stir in the split peas, potatoes, bay leaf, vegetable broth, and water. Bring the mixture to a boil.
4. Reduce the heat to a simmer, cover, and cook for 40-45 minutes or until the split peas are tender, stirring occasionally.
5. Remove the bay leaf and discard it.
6. Using an immersion blender or a regular blender, puree the soup until smooth. If using a regular blender, be sure to cool the soup slightly before blending.

7. Return the soup to the pot, and reheat if necessary.

8. Season with salt and pepper to taste.

9. Serve hot, garnished with fresh parsley if desired.

Useful Tip: To add an extra layer of flavor, consider adding a dash of smoked paprika or a squeeze of lemon juice before serving. This Vegan Split Pea Soup is not only delicious but also suitable for a gallbladder diet. Enjoy!

Nutritional Values: Calories: 220 kcal | Fat: 2g | Protein: 12g | Carbs: 40g | Net carbs: 30g | Fiber: 10g | Cholesterol: 0mg | Sodium: 840mg | Potassium: 590mg

Red Lentil and Spinach Soup

Serving: 4 | Prep time: 10 minutes | Cook time: 25 minutes

Ingredients:

- 8 oz (227g) red lentils
- 2 oz (57g) onion, finely chopped
- 2 oz (57g) carrots, diced
- 2 oz (57g) celery, diced
- 2 cloves garlic, minced
- 1 tsp olive oil
- 32 oz (960ml) vegetable broth
- 16 oz (480ml) water
- 2 oz (57g) fresh spinach, chopped
- 1 tsp ground cumin
- 1/2 tsp ground coriander
- Salt and pepper to taste
- Fresh cilantro for garnish (optional)

Directions:

1. Rinse the red lentils under cold water and set them aside.

2. In a large pot, heat the olive oil over medium heat. Add the onions, garlic, carrots, and celery. Sauté until the vegetables start to soften, about 5 minutes.

3. Stir in the ground cumin and ground coriander, and cook for another 2 minutes until fragrant.

4. Add the red lentils, vegetable broth, and water. Bring the mixture to a boil.

5. Reduce the heat to a simmer, cover, and cook for 20-25 minutes, or until the lentils are tender, stirring occasionally.

6. Stir in the chopped spinach and cook for an additional 2-3 minutes until wilted.

7. Season with salt and pepper to taste.

8. Serve hot, garnished with fresh cilantro if desired.

Useful Tip: For a touch of acidity and brightness, consider adding a squeeze of fresh lemon juice to your individual serving just before enjoying this Red Lentil and Spinach Soup. It's a flavorful and gallbladder-friendly delight!

Nutritional Values: Calories: 220 kcal | Fat: 2g | Protein: 15g | Carbs: 38g | Net carbs: 30g | Fiber: 8g | Cholesterol: 0mg | Sodium: 980mg | Potassium: 640mg

Zucchini and Basil Soup

Serving: 4 | Prep time: 15 minutes | Cook time: 25 minutes

Ingredients:

- 12 oz (340g) zucchini, sliced
- 4 oz (113g) onion, chopped
- 2 cloves garlic, minced
- 1 tsp olive oil
- 32 oz (960ml) vegetable broth
- 1 oz (28g) fresh basil leaves
- 4 oz (113g) potatoes, peeled and diced
- Salt and pepper to taste
- 2 oz (57g) plain Greek yogurt
- Fresh basil leaves for garnish (optional)

Directions:

1. In a large pot, heat the olive oil over medium heat. Add the chopped onions and garlic, and sauté until they

become translucent, about 3-4 minutes.

2. Add the sliced zucchini and potatoes to the pot and continue to sauté for another 3-4 minutes.

3. Pour in the vegetable broth and bring the mixture to a boil.

4. Reduce the heat to a simmer, cover, and cook for 15-20 minutes, or until the vegetables are tender.

5. Remove the pot from heat, and stir in the fresh basil leaves.

6. Use an immersion blender to carefully puree the soup until smooth. If you don't have an immersion blender, allow the soup to cool slightly and puree it in batches using a regular blender.

7. Return the pureed soup to the pot, and season with salt and pepper to taste.

8. Serve hot, garnished with a dollop of plain Greek yogurt and fresh basil leaves if desired.

Useful Tip: To make this Zucchini and Basil Soup even creamier and dairy-free, substitute plain Greek yogurt with a dollop of unsweetened coconut yogurt or almond yogurt before serving. Enjoy this delightful and gallbladder-friendly soup!

Nutritional Values: Calories: 120 kcal | Fat: 2g | Protein: 6g | Carbs: 23g | Net carbs: 15g | Fiber: 8g | Cholesterol: 0mg | Sodium: 720mg | Potassium: 740mg

Pea and Mint Soup

Serving: 4 | Prep time: 10 minutes | Cook time: 20 minutes

Ingredients:

- 12 oz (340g) frozen green peas
- 1 oz (28g) onion, chopped
- 1 oz (28g) celery, chopped
- 1 oz (28g) leek, chopped
- 1 tsp olive oil

- 32 oz (960ml) vegetable broth
- 2 oz (57g) fresh mint leaves
- Salt and pepper to taste
- 2 oz (57g) plain Greek yogurt
- Fresh mint leaves for garnish (optional)

Directions:

1. In a large pot, heat the olive oil over medium heat. Add the chopped onion, celery, and leek, and sauté until they become translucent, about 3-4 minutes.

2. Add the frozen green peas to the pot and continue to sauté for another 3-4 minutes.

3. Pour in the vegetable broth and bring the mixture to a boil.

4. Reduce the heat to a simmer, cover, and cook for 15 minutes, or until the peas are tender.

5. Remove the pot from heat, and stir in the fresh mint leaves.

6. Use an immersion blender to carefully puree the soup until smooth. If you don't have an immersion blender, allow the soup to cool slightly and puree it in batches using a regular blender.

7. Return the pureed soup to the pot, and season with salt and pepper to taste.

8. Serve hot, garnished with a dollop of plain Greek yogurt and fresh mint leaves if desired.

Useful Tip: For a dairy-free option, replace the plain Greek yogurt with a spoonful of coconut cream or almond-based yogurt. Enjoy this light and gallbladder-friendly Pea and Mint Soup!

Nutritional Values: Calories: 90 kcal | Fat: 2g | Protein: 6g | Carbs: 15g | Net carbs: 10g | Fiber: 5g | Cholesterol: 0mg | Sodium: 720mg | Potassium: 550mg

Asparagus and Potato Soup

Serving: 4 | Prep time: 15 minutes | Cook time: 25 minutes

Ingredients:

- 8 oz (227g) asparagus spears, trimmed and chopped
- 8 oz (227g) potatoes, peeled and diced

- 1 oz (28g) leek, chopped
- 1 oz (28g) onion, chopped
- 1 tsp olive oil

- 32 oz (960ml) vegetable broth
- 1 tsp lemon juice
- Salt and pepper to taste
- 2 oz (57g) plain Greek yogurt (optional, for garnish)
- Fresh dill leaves for garnish (optional)

Directions:

1. In a large pot, heat the olive oil over medium heat. Add the chopped leek and onion, and sauté until they become translucent, about 3-4 minutes.
2. Add the diced potatoes and chopped asparagus to the pot, and sauté for another 3-4 minutes.
3. Pour in the vegetable broth and bring the mixture to a boil.
4. Reduce the heat to a simmer, cover, and cook for 15-20 minutes, or until the vegetables are tender.
5. Remove the pot from heat and use an immersion blender to carefully puree the soup until smooth. If you don't have an immersion blender, allow the soup to cool slightly and puree it in batches using a regular blender.
6. Stir in the lemon juice, and season with salt and pepper to taste.
7. Serve hot, garnished with a dollop of plain Greek yogurt and fresh dill leaves if desired.

Useful Tip: For a creamier texture, blend in 2 ounces (57g) of plain Greek yogurt before serving. Enjoy this nutritious Asparagus and Potato Soup as a satisfying and gallbladder-friendly dish!

Nutritional Values: Calories: 110 kcal | Fat: 1g | Protein: 4g | Carbs: 23g | Net carbs: 15g | Fiber: 8g | Cholesterol: 0mg | Sodium: 800mg | Potassium: 580mg

Cabbage and White Bean Soup

Serving: 4 | Prep time: 15 minutes | Cook time: 25 minutes

Ingredients:

- 8 oz (227g) cabbage, shredded
- 8 oz (227g) canned white beans, drained and rinsed
- 4 oz (113g) carrots, diced
- 4 oz (113g) celery, diced
- 4 oz (113g) onion, chopped
- 1 clove garlic, minced
- 1 tsp olive oil
- 32 oz (960ml) vegetable broth
- 1 tsp dried thyme
- Salt and pepper to taste
- 2 tbsp fresh parsley, chopped (for garnish)
- Lemon wedges (for garnish, optional)

Directions:

1. In a large pot, heat the olive oil over medium heat. Add the chopped onion and garlic and sauté until fragrant, about 2-3 minutes.
2. Add the diced carrots and celery to the pot, and sauté for another 3-4 minutes.
3. Stir in the shredded cabbage and sauté until it begins to wilt, about 2 minutes.
4. Pour in the vegetable broth and bring the mixture to a boil.
5. Reduce the heat to a simmer, cover, and cook for 15-20 minutes, or until the vegetables are tender.
6. Add the drained and rinsed white beans and dried thyme to the pot. Cook for an additional 5 minutes until heated through.
7. Season with salt and pepper to taste.
8. Serve hot, garnished with chopped fresh parsley and a lemon wedge if desired.

Useful Tip: To add an extra zing to your soup, squeeze a fresh lemon wedge over each serving just before enjoying. This Cabbage and White Bean Soup is both delicious and gallbladder-friendly!

Nutritional Values: Calories: 120 kcal | Fat: 2g | Protein: 6g | Carbs: 22g | Net carbs: 15g | Fiber: 7g | Cholesterol: 0mg | Sodium: 850mg | Potassium: 560mg

Beet and Carrot Soup

Serving: 4 | Prep time: 15 minutes | Cook time: 30 minutes

Ingredients:

- 8 oz (227g) beets, peeled and chopped
- 8 oz (227g) carrots, peeled and chopped
- 4 oz (113g) onion, chopped
- 2 cloves garlic, minced
- 1 tsp olive oil
- 32 oz (960ml) vegetable broth
- 1 tsp ground cumin
- Salt and pepper to taste
- 2 tbsp plain Greek yogurt (for garnish)
- Fresh dill or parsley (for garnish)

Directions:

1. In a large pot, heat the olive oil over medium heat. Add the chopped onion and garlic and sauté until fragrant, about 2-3 minutes.
2. Add the chopped beets and carrots to the pot and sauté for another 5 minutes.
3. Pour in the vegetable broth and bring the mixture to a boil.
4. Reduce the heat to a simmer, cover, and cook for 20-25 minutes, or until the vegetables are tender.
5. Using an immersion blender or a regular blender, carefully puree the soup until smooth.
6. Stir in the ground cumin and season with salt and pepper to taste.
7. Serve hot, garnished with a dollop of plain Greek yogurt and fresh dill or parsley.

Useful Tip: For a creamier texture, you can add a splash of low-fat milk or dairy-free milk alternative when blending the soup. This Beet and Carrot Soup is a nutritious and gallbladder-friendly option for a comforting meal. Enjoy!

Nutritional Values: Calories: 120 kcal | Fat: 2g | Protein: 4g | Carbs: 22g | Net carbs: 16g | Fiber: 6g | Cholesterol: 0mg | Sodium: 900mg | Potassium: 680mg

SMOOTHIES

Banana Berry Bliss

Serving: 4 | Prep time: 10 minutes | Cook time: 0 minutes

Ingredients:

- 12 oz (340g) mixed berries (strawberries, blueberries, raspberries)
- 2 ripe bananas
- 6 oz (170g) plain Greek yogurt
- 1 tbsp honey
- 1 tsp vanilla extract
- 4 oz (120ml) unsweetened almond milk
- 1 tbsp chia seeds
- Fresh mint leaves (for garnish)

Directions:

1. Wash and dry the mixed berries. If using strawberries, remove the stems.
2. Peel the ripe bananas and cut them into chunks.
3. In a blender, combine the mixed berries, bananas, plain Greek yogurt, honey, vanilla extract, and unsweetened almond milk.
4. Blend until the mixture is smooth and well combined.
5. Transfer the blended mixture to a bowl and stir in the chia seeds.
6. Cover the bowl and refrigerate for at least 1 hour or until the chia seeds have absorbed some of the liquid and the mixture has thickened.
7. Before serving, garnish with fresh mint leaves.
8. Enjoy this delightful and gallbladder-friendly Banana Berry Bliss as a healthy breakfast or snack!

Useful Tip: You can customize this recipe by adding a handful of spinach or kale for an extra nutritional boost without altering the delightful flavor.

Nutritional Values: Calories: 150 kcal | Fat: 2g | Protein: 6g | Carbs: 30g | Net carbs: 20g | Fiber: 10g | Cholesterol: 5mg | Sodium: 40mg | Potassium: 340mg

Mango Tango Smoothie

Serving: 4 | Prep time: 5 minutes | Cook time: 0 minutes

Ingredients:

- 16 oz (450g) frozen mango chunks
- 1 ripe banana
- 8 oz (240ml) unsweetened coconut milk
- 4 oz (120ml) plain Greek yogurt
- 1 tbsp honey
- 1 tsp freshly squeezed lime juice
- 1/2 tsp vanilla extract
- 8 oz (240ml) ice cubes

Directions:

1. In a blender, combine the frozen mango chunks, ripe banana, unsweetened coconut milk, plain Greek yogurt, honey, freshly squeezed lime juice, vanilla extract, and ice cubes.
2. Blend until the mixture is smooth and creamy.
3. Taste the smoothie and adjust sweetness by adding more honey if desired.
4. Pour into glasses and serve immediately.
5. Enjoy this refreshing and gallbladder-friendly Mango Tango Smoothie as a nutritious breakfast or snack!

Useful Tip: For an extra burst of flavor and nutrients, consider adding a handful of spinach or kale to the blender to create a vibrant green Mango Tango Smoothie.

Nutritional Values: Calories: 150 kcal | Fat: 2g | Protein: 3g | Carbs: 35g | Net carbs: 28g | Fiber: 7g | Cholesterol: 5mg | Sodium: 30mg | Potassium: 400mg

Green Detox Smoothie

Serving: 4 | Prep time: 10 minutes | Cook time: 0 minutes

Ingredients:

- 12 oz (340g) fresh spinach leaves
- 2 ripe bananas
- 8 oz (240ml) unsweetened almond milk
- 1/2 cucumber, peeled and chopped
- 1 green apple, cored and chopped
- 1/2 avocado, peeled and pitted
- 1 tbsp freshly squeezed lemon juice
- 1 tsp honey (optional)
- 8 oz (240ml) ice cubes

Directions:

1. In a blender, combine the fresh spinach leaves, ripe bananas, unsweetened almond milk, chopped cucumber, chopped green apple, peeled and pitted avocado, freshly squeezed lemon juice, and honey (if desired).
2. Add the ice cubes to the blender to make the smoothie cold and refreshing.
3. Blend until all the ingredients are well combined and the smoothie is creamy.
4. Taste the smoothie and adjust sweetness by adding more honey if needed.
5. Pour into glasses and garnish with a slice of cucumber or a lemon wheel, if desired.
6. Enjoy this Green Detox Smoothie packed with nutrients and suitable for a gallbladder-friendly diet!

Useful Tip: To make your Green Detox Smoothie even more refreshing, consider using frozen banana slices instead of fresh ones, which will add a natural sweetness and an extra chill to your drink.

Nutritional Values: Calories: 150 kcal | Fat: 5g | Protein: 3g | Carbs: 27g | Net carbs: 18g | Fiber: 9g | Cholesterol: 0mg | Sodium: 140mg | Potassium: 650mg

Pineapple Coconut Delight

Serving: 4 | Prep time: 10 minutes | Cook time: 0 minutes

Ingredients:

- 16 oz (450g) fresh pineapple chunks
- 6 oz (170g) unsweetened shredded coconut
- 8 oz (240ml) unsweetened coconut milk
- 2 tbsp honey (optional)
- 1 tsp pure vanilla extract
- 8 oz (240ml) ice cubes

Directions:

1. In a blender, combine the fresh pineapple chunks, unsweetened shredded coconut, unsweetened coconut milk, honey (if desired), and pure vanilla extract.
2. Add the ice cubes to the blender to make the smoothie cold and refreshing.
3. Blend until all the ingredients are well combined, and the smoothie is creamy.
4. Taste the smoothie and adjust sweetness by adding more honey if needed.
5. Pour into glasses and garnish with a pineapple slice or a sprinkle of shredded coconut, if desired.
6. Enjoy this Pineapple Coconut Delight, a tropical treat that's suitable for a gallbladder-friendly diet!

Useful Tip: For an even creamier texture, you can use frozen pineapple chunks instead of fresh ones. This will also enhance the chilling effect of your Pineapple Coconut Delight without the need for additional ice.

Nutritional Values: Calories: 350 kcal | Fat: 22g | Protein: 3g | Carbs: 38g | Net carbs: 30g | Fiber: 8g | Cholesterol: 0mg | Sodium: 20mg | Potassium: 400mg

Avocado and Spinach Smoothie

Serving: 4 | Prep time: 5 minutes | Cook time: 0 minutes

Ingredients:

- 2 ripe avocados, peeled and pitted (about 14 oz or 400g)
- 32 oz (960ml) unsweetened almond milk
- 6 oz (170g) fresh spinach leaves
- 2 tbsp lemon juice
- 2 tbsp honey (optional)
- 1 tsp pure vanilla extract
- 8 oz (480ml) ice cubes

Directions:

1. In a blender, combine the ripe avocados, unsweetened almond milk, fresh spinach leaves, lemon juice, honey (if desired), and pure vanilla extract.
2. Add the ice cubes to the blender for a refreshing chill.
3. Blend until the ingredients are thoroughly combined, and the smoothie is creamy and vibrant green.
4. Taste the smoothie and adjust sweetness by adding more honey if needed.
5. Pour into glasses, garnish with a spinach leaf or a slice of avocado, if desired.
6. Enjoy this Avocado and Spinach Smoothie, a nutritious and gallbladder-friendly delight!

Useful Tip: If you prefer an even thicker smoothie, you can use frozen avocado chunks instead of fresh avocados. This will provide the same creaminess without diluting the flavor with extra ice.

Nutritional Values: Calories: 250 kcal | Fat: 17g | Protein: 4g | Carbs: 24g | Net carbs: 12g | Fiber: 12g | Cholesterol: 0mg | Sodium: 220mg | Potassium: 900mg

Blueberry Almond Protein Smoothie

Serving: 4 | Prep time: 5 minutes | Cook time: 0 minutes

Ingredients:

- 12 oz (340g) frozen blueberries
- 4 oz (115g) unsweetened almond butter
- 32 oz (960ml) unsweetened almond milk
- 2 oz (57g) unsweetened almond protein powder
- 2 tbsp honey (optional)
- 1 tsp almond extract
- 8 oz (480ml) ice cubes

Directions:

1. In a blender, add the frozen blueberries, unsweetened almond butter, unsweetened almond milk, unsweetened almond protein powder, honey (if desired), almond extract, and ice cubes.
2. Blend until the ingredients are well combined and the smoothie is creamy and purple.
3. Taste the smoothie and adjust sweetness by adding more honey if needed.
4. Pour into glasses, garnish with a few fresh blueberries or a drizzle of almond butter, if desired.
5. Enjoy the Blueberry Almond Protein Smoothie, a delicious and gallbladder-friendly protein boost!

Useful Tip: For an extra nutritional boost, consider adding a handful of fresh spinach or kale to this smoothie. It'll increase the fiber and nutrient content without compromising the delicious taste.

Nutritional Values: Calories: 250 kcal | Fat: 15g | Protein: 10g | Carbs: 25g | Net carbs: 18g | Fiber: 7g | Cholesterol: 0mg | Sodium: 280mg | Potassium: 550mg

Peachy Keen Smoothie

Serving: 4 | Prep time: 5 minutes | Cook time: 0 minutes

Ingredients:

- 12 oz (340g) frozen peaches
- 4 oz (115g) Greek yogurt
- 32 oz (960ml) unsweetened almond milk
- 2 oz (57g) vanilla protein powder
- 2 tbsp honey (optional)
- 1 tsp vanilla extract
- 8 oz (480ml) ice cubes

Directions:

1. In a blender, combine the frozen peaches, Greek yogurt, unsweetened almond milk, vanilla protein powder, honey (if desired), vanilla extract, and ice cubes.
2. Blend until the mixture is smooth and creamy, with a delightful peachy color.
3. Taste the smoothie and adjust sweetness with additional honey, if needed.
4. Pour into glasses and serve immediately.
5. Sip on the Peachy Keen Smoothie for a gallbladder-friendly and refreshing treat!

Useful Tip: To make this smoothie even more nutrient-rich, add a handful of fresh spinach or kale. It won't alter the delicious peach flavor but will give you an extra boost of vitamins and minerals. Enjoy your healthy, green Peachy Keen Smoothie!

Nutritional Values: Calories: 220 kcal | Fat: 5g | Protein: 18g | Carbs: 27g | Net carbs: 20g | Fiber: 7g | Cholesterol: 5mg | Sodium: 260mg | Potassium: 550mg

Cucumber Mint Cooler

Serving: 4 | Prep time: 10 minutes | Cook time: 0 minutes

Ingredients:

- 20 oz (570g) cucumber, peeled and diced
- 2 oz (57g) fresh mint leaves
- 16 oz (480ml) cold water
- 2 oz (57g) fresh lime juice
- 1 oz (30ml) honey (optional)
- 8 oz (480ml) ice cubes

Directions:

1. In a blender, combine the diced cucumber, fresh mint leaves, cold water, fresh lime juice, and honey (if desired).
2. Blend until the mixture is smooth and the mint leaves are finely chopped.
3. Taste the cooler and adjust sweetness with additional honey, if needed.
4. Add the ice cubes to the blender and pulse until the ice is crushed and the cooler is icy cold.
5. Pour the Cucumber Mint Cooler into glasses.
6. Garnish with fresh mint leaves and cucumber slices.
7. Sip and savor this refreshing and gallbladder-friendly beverage!

Useful Tip: For an extra twist, add a splash of sparkling water to each glass before serving to make it effervescent and even more refreshing. Enjoy your cool and revitalizing Cucumber Mint Cooler!

Nutritional Values: Calories: 30 kcal | Fat: 0g | Protein: 0g | Carbs: 8g | Net carbs: 7g | Fiber: 1g | Cholesterol: 0mg | Sodium: 10mg | Potassium: 60mg

Начало формы

Carrot Cake Smoothie

Serving: 4 | Prep time: 10 minutes | Cook time: 0 minutes

Ingredients:

- 12 oz (340g) carrots, peeled and chopped
- 6 oz (170g) ripe bananas, sliced
- 4 oz (113g) Greek yogurt
- 2 oz (57g) rolled oats
- 16 oz (480ml) unsweetened almond milk
- 2 oz (57g) walnuts, chopped
- 1 tsp ground cinnamon
- 1/2 tsp ground nutmeg
- 1/2 tsp vanilla extract
- 2 tbsp honey (optional, for sweetness)
- 8 oz (480ml) ice cubes

Directions:

1. In a blender, combine the chopped carrots, sliced bananas, Greek yogurt, rolled oats, unsweetened almond milk, chopped walnuts, ground cinnamon, ground nutmeg, vanilla extract, and honey (if using).
2. Blend until smooth and creamy.
3. Add the ice cubes to the blender and blend again until the smoothie is thick and icy.
4. Pour the Carrot Cake Smoothie into glasses.
5. Garnish with a sprinkle of cinnamon and a few chopped walnuts if desired.
6. Indulge in the delightful flavors of carrot cake in a refreshing smoothie form!

Useful Tip: For an extra touch, top the smoothie with a dollop of Greek yogurt and a drizzle of honey. This smoothie captures all the essence of carrot cake without the guilt, making it a perfect treat for any time of the day. Enjoy the sweet and spicy goodness of this Carrot Cake Smoothie!

Nutritional Values: Calories: 180 kcal | Fat: 7g | Protein: 6g | Carbs: 27g | Net carbs: 20g | Fiber: 7g | Cholesterol: 0mg | Sodium: 180mg | Potassium: 460mg

Cherry Almond Bliss

Serving: 4 | Prep time: 5 minutes | Cook time: 0 minutes

Ingredients:

- 12 oz (340g) frozen cherries
- 4 oz (113g) plain Greek yogurt
- 8 oz (227g) unsweetened almond milk
- 2 oz (57g) almonds
- 1 tbsp honey (optional, for sweetness)
- 1 tsp almond extract
- 1/2 tsp vanilla extract
- 8 oz (480ml) ice cubes

Directions:

1. In a blender, combine the frozen cherries, plain Greek yogurt, unsweetened almond milk, almonds, honey (if using), almond extract, and vanilla extract.
2. Blend until smooth and creamy.
3. Add the ice cubes to the blender and blend again until the smoothie is thick and frosty.
4. Pour the Cherry Almond Bliss into glasses.
5. Garnish with a few whole almonds or a fresh cherry on the rim of each glass if desired.
6. Relish in the delightful combination of cherries and almonds in this blissful smoothie!

Useful Tip: To intensify the almond flavor, you can add a small pinch of ground cinnamon to the blender. This Cherry Almond Bliss is a perfect way to satisfy your sweet cravings without compromising on your dietary needs. Enjoy the indulgent taste of cherries and almonds in every sip!

Nutritional Values: Calories: 180 kcal | Fat: 8g | Protein: 6g | Carbs: 20g | Net carbs: 16g | Fiber: 4g | Cholesterol: 0mg | Sodium: 90mg | Potassium: 320mg

Strawberry Kiwi Quencher

Serving: 4 | Prep time: 10 minutes | Cook time: 0 minutes

Ingredients:

- 12 oz (340g) fresh strawberries, hulled
- 8 oz (227g) ripe kiwi, peeled and sliced
- 2 oz (57g) honey (adjust to taste)
- 4 oz (113g) plain Greek yogurt
- 8 oz (227g) cold water
- 1 tsp lemon juice
- 1/2 tsp vanilla extract
- 8 oz (480ml) ice cubes

Directions:

1. Place the fresh strawberries, ripe kiwi, honey, plain Greek yogurt, cold water, lemon juice, and vanilla extract in a blender.
2. Blend until the mixture is smooth and the fruits are fully pureed.
3. Add the ice cubes and blend again until the smoothie is well chilled.
4. Taste the Strawberry Kiwi Quencher and adjust the sweetness with more honey if desired.
5. Pour the refreshing smoothie into glasses.
6. Garnish with a strawberry slice and a kiwi wheel on the rim of each glass, if desired.
7. Sip and savor this delightful quencher!

Useful Tip: If you prefer a thicker consistency, you can add more ice cubes or a small handful of frozen strawberries before blending. This Strawberry Kiwi Quencher is a perfect way to cool down on a hot day while adhering to your dietary requirements. Enjoy the vibrant flavors of strawberries and kiwis in every sip!

Nutritional Values: Calories: 110 kcal | Fat: 1g | Protein: 4g | Carbs: 25g | Net carbs: 22g | Fiber: 3g | Cholesterol: 2mg | Sodium: 25mg | Potassium: 330mg

Tropical Turmeric Twist

Serving: 4 | Prep time: 5 minutes | Cook time: 0 minutes

Ingredients:

- 8 oz (227g) frozen mango chunks
- 6 oz (170g) frozen pineapple chunks
- 2 ripe bananas
- 1 tsp ground turmeric
- 1/2 tsp ground ginger
- 1/2 tsp ground cinnamon
- 4 oz (113g) plain Greek yogurt
- 16 oz (473ml) unsweetened coconut water
- 1 tsp honey (optional, adjust to taste)
- Ice cubes (optional)
- Fresh mint leaves for garnish (optional)

Directions:

1. Place the frozen mango chunks, frozen pineapple chunks, ripe bananas, ground turmeric, ground ginger, ground cinnamon, plain Greek yogurt, and unsweetened coconut water in a blender.
2. Blend until all the ingredients are well combined and the mixture is smooth.
3. Taste the Tropical Turmeric Twist and add honey if you prefer it sweeter.
4. If you want a colder drink, you can add ice cubes and blend again until well incorporated.
5. Pour the refreshing Tropical Turmeric Twist into glasses.
6. Garnish with fresh mint leaves if desired.
7. Sip and savor the tropical flavors with a twist of turmeric!

Useful Tip: For a creamier texture and added protein, you can use coconut milk or almond milk instead of coconut water. Enjoy this Tropical Turmeric Twist as a nutritious and delicious way to start your day or as a refreshing pick-me-up in the afternoon!

Nutritional Values: Calories: 150 kcal | Fat: 1g | Protein: 4g | Carbs: 35g | Net carbs: 27g | Fiber: 8g | Cholesterol: 2mg | Sodium: 100mg | Potassium: 720mg

Raspberry Coconut Dream

Serving: 4 | Prep time: 5 minutes | Cook time: 0 minutes

Ingredients:

- 6 oz (170g) fresh raspberries
- 4 oz (113g) unsweetened shredded coconut
- 16 oz (473ml) unsweetened coconut milk
- 1 ripe banana
- 2 tbsp honey (adjust to taste)
- 1 tsp vanilla extract
- 8 oz (237ml) water
- Ice cubes (optional)

Directions:

1. Combine the fresh raspberries, unsweetened shredded coconut, unsweetened coconut milk, ripe banana, honey, vanilla extract, and water in a blender.
2. Blend until the mixture is smooth and all ingredients are well combined.
3. Taste the Raspberry Coconut Dream and adjust the sweetness with additional honey if desired.
4. If you prefer your smoothie extra cold, add some ice cubes to the blender and blend again until smooth.
5. Pour the Raspberry Coconut Dream into glasses.
6. Garnish with a few fresh raspberries or a sprinkle of shredded coconut if you like.
7. Sip and savor the delightful, tropical flavors of this dreamy smoothie!

Useful Tip: For an even creamier texture and more coconut flavor, you can use canned coconut milk instead of unsweetened coconut milk. This Raspberry Coconut Dream is a wonderful way to treat yourself to a taste of the tropics while staying within your dietary guidelines. Enjoy the refreshing and healthy goodness!

Nutritional Values: Calories: 280 kcal | Fat: 20g | Protein: 3g | Carbs: 25g | Net carbs: 17g | Fiber: 8g | Cholesterol: 0mg | Sodium: 15mg | Potassium: 372mg

Spinach and Apple Detox

Serving: 4 | Prep time: 10 minutes | Cook time: 0 minutes

Ingredients:

- 8 oz (227g) fresh baby spinach
- 2 medium apples, cored and sliced (skin on)
- 1 cucumber, peeled and chopped
- 1 lemon, peeled and seeded
- 1-inch (2.5 cm) piece of fresh ginger, peeled
- 16 oz (473ml) cold water
- Ice cubes (optional)
- Fresh mint leaves for garnish (optional)

Directions:

1. Place the fresh baby spinach, sliced apples, chopped cucumber, peeled lemon, and peeled ginger in a blender.
2. Pour in the cold water to help with blending.
3. Blend until you achieve a smooth consistency, adding more water if needed to reach your desired thickness.
4. If you prefer your detox drink extra cold, add a handful of ice cubes to the blender and blend again until smooth.
5. Taste the Spinach and Apple Detox and adjust the flavor by adding more lemon if desired.
6. Pour the detox drink into glasses.
7. Garnish with fresh mint leaves for a refreshing touch.
8. Sip and enjoy the revitalizing flavors of this nutritious detox drink!

Useful Tip: To make this detox even more refreshing, you can chill your glasses in the freezer before serving. This Spinach and Apple Detox is a great way to boost your nutrient intake and help your body feel its best. Enjoy this healthy and delicious drink!

Nutritional Values: Calories: 65 kcal | Fat: 0g | Protein: 1g | Carbs: 16g | Net carbs: 10g | Fiber: 6g | Cholesterol: 0mg | Sodium: 30mg | Potassium: 389mg

Mint Chocolate Chip Delight

Serving: 4 | Prep time: 10 minutes | Cook time: 0 minutes

Ingredients:

- 8 oz (227g) frozen spinach
- 1 medium ripe banana
- 2 tbsp unsweetened cocoa powder
- 2 tbsp almond butter
- 1/2 tsp peppermint extract
- 16 oz (473ml) unsweetened almond milk
- 1-2 tbsp dark chocolate chips (70% cocoa or higher)
- Ice cubes (optional)
- Fresh mint leaves for garnish (optional)

Directions:

1. In a blender, combine the frozen spinach, ripe banana, unsweetened cocoa powder, almond butter, and peppermint extract.
2. Pour in the unsweetened almond milk.
3. Blend until the mixture is smooth and creamy. If you prefer a colder drink, you can add ice cubes at this point and blend again.
4. Taste the Mint Chocolate Chip Delight and adjust the sweetness or mint flavor as needed.
5. If you'd like some chocolatey crunch, stir in 1-2 tablespoons of dark chocolate chips.
6. Pour the delightful green smoothie into glasses.
7. Garnish with fresh mint leaves for a burst of freshness.
8. Sip and savor the blissful combination of mint and chocolate in this healthy and indulgent smoothie.

Useful Tip: For an extra creamy texture and an even cooler Mint Chocolate Chip Delight, use a frozen banana instead of a ripe one, and skip the ice cubes. This will make your smoothie wonderfully thick and frosty. Enjoy this guilt-free dessert-inspired treat!

Nutritional Values: Calories: 160 kcal | Fat: 7g | Protein: 4g | Carbs: 24g | Net carbs: 16g | Fiber: 8g | Cholesterol: 0mg | Sodium: 205mg | Potassium: 583mg

Chia Berry Blast

Serving: 4 | Prep time: 10 minutes | Cook time: 0 minutes

Ingredients:

- 2 oz (57g) chia seeds
- 16 oz (473ml) unsweetened almond milk
- 4 oz (140g) mixed berries (strawberries, raspberries)
- 2 tbsp honey or maple syrup (optional for sweetness)
- 1 tsp vanilla extract
- Fresh berries and mint leaves for garnish (optional)

Directions:

1. In a mixing bowl, combine the chia seeds and unsweetened almond milk.
2. Add the mixed berries, sweetener (if using), and vanilla extract to the bowl.
3. Mix all the ingredients thoroughly.
4. Cover the bowl and refrigerate it for at least 2 hours or overnight, allowing the chia seeds to absorb the liquid and create a thick, pudding-like texture.
5. Stir the Chia Berry Blast well before serving to evenly distribute the chia seeds.
6. Divide the chia pudding into serving glasses.
7. Garnish with fresh berries and mint leaves for a burst of color and flavor.
8. Enjoy this delightful and nutritious chia seed pudding!

Useful Tip: Feel free to customize your Chia Berry Blast by using your favorite mix of berries or adjusting the sweetness level to your preference. This make-ahead breakfast or snack is a fantastic source of fiber and healthy fats, making it a great addition to your gallbladder-friendly diet. Enjoy!

Nutritional Values: Calories: 150 kcal | Fat: 7g | Protein: 3g | Carbs: 19g | Net carbs: 11g | Fiber: 8g | Cholesterol: 0mg | Sodium: 92mg | Potassium: 115mg

Vanilla Fig Smoothie

Serving: 4 | Prep time: 10 minutes | Cook time: 0 minutes

Ingredients:

- 8 oz (227g) fresh figs, stems removed and quartered
- 16 oz (473ml) unsweetened almond milk
- 2 tbsp almond butter
- 1 tsp pure vanilla extract
- 1/2 tsp ground cinnamon
- 1/2 tsp honey or maple syrup (optional for added sweetness)
- Ice cubes (optional)
- Fresh fig slices and a sprinkle of cinnamon for garnish (optional)

Directions:

1. Place the fresh figs, unsweetened almond milk, almond butter, vanilla extract, ground cinnamon, and sweetener (if using) in a blender.
2. If you prefer a colder smoothie, you can add a few ice cubes to the blender as well.
3. Blend all the ingredients until the mixture is smooth and creamy, usually for about 1-2 minutes.
4. Taste the smoothie and adjust the sweetness or cinnamon level as needed.
5. Pour the Vanilla Fig Smoothie into serving glasses.
6. Garnish with fresh fig slices and a sprinkle of cinnamon for a delightful presentation.
7. Enjoy this unique and gallbladder-friendly smoothie!

Useful Tip: Fresh figs are the star of this smoothie, providing natural sweetness and a unique flavor. Adjust the sweetness to your preference, keeping in mind that honey or maple syrup can be omitted if you prefer a lower-sugar option. This smoothie is an excellent source of fiber and healthy fats, making it a nutritious addition to your gallbladder diet. Enjoy!

Nutritional Values: Calories: 125 kcal | Fat: 8g | Protein: 3g | Carbs: 13g | Net carbs: 9g | Fiber: 4g | Cholesterol: 0mg | Sodium: 164mg | Potassium: 200mg

Watermelon Cucumber Cooler

Serving: 4 | Prep time: 10 minutes | Cook time: 0 minutes

Ingredients:

- 24 oz (680g) fresh watermelon, cubed
- 8 oz (227g) cucumber, peeled and chopped
- 4 oz (118ml) coconut water
- Juice of 1 lime
- 1 tsp honey or maple syrup (optional, for added sweetness)
- Fresh mint leaves for garnish
- Ice cubes (optional)

Directions:

1. Place the fresh watermelon cubes, chopped cucumber, coconut water, lime juice, and sweetener (if using) in a blender.
2. If you prefer a colder cooler, you can add a few ice cubes to the blender as well.
3. Blend all the ingredients until you have a smooth and refreshing mixture, which should take about 1-2 minutes.
4. Taste the cooler and adjust the sweetness or lime juice according to your preference.
5. Pour the Watermelon Cucumber Cooler into serving glasses.

6. Garnish with fresh mint leaves for a burst of flavor and a touch of elegance.

7. Sip and enjoy this gallbladder-friendly cooler on a hot day!

Useful Tip: This Watermelon Cucumber Cooler is not only hydrating but also packed with vitamins and antioxidants. The honey or maple syrup can be omitted if you prefer a lower-sugar option, as the natural sweetness of the watermelon often suffices. Enjoy this refreshing drink to stay cool and keep your gallbladder diet on track!

Nutritional Values: Calories: 45 kcal | Fat: 0.5g | Protein: 1g | Carbs: 11g | Net carbs: 8g | Fiber: 3g | Cholesterol: 0mg | Sodium: 43mg | Potassium: 314mg

DESSERTS

Banana-Oatmeal Cookies

Serving: 4 | Prep time: 10 minutes | Cook time: 15 minutes

Ingredients:

- 4 oz (113g) ripe bananas, mashed
- 4 oz (113g) rolled oats
- 1 oz (28g) almond butter
- 1 oz (28g) honey or maple syrup
- 1 tsp vanilla extract
- 1/2 tsp ground cinnamon
- 1/4 tsp salt
- 1 oz (28g) dark chocolate chips (optional)
- 1 oz (28g) chopped nuts of your choice (optional)

Directions:

1. Preheat your oven to 350°F (175°C).
2. In a mixing bowl, combine the mashed bananas, rolled oats, almond butter, honey or maple syrup, vanilla extract, ground cinnamon, and a pinch of salt.
3. If you prefer, you can add dark chocolate chips or chopped nuts to the mixture for extra flavor and texture.
4. Stir the ingredients until well combined.
5. Line a baking sheet with parchment paper or lightly grease it.
6. Using a spoon or your hands, form small cookie-shaped portions from the mixture and place them on the baking sheet.
7. Flatten each cookie with a fork or the back of a spoon.
8. Bake in the preheated oven for about 15 minutes or until the cookies turn golden brown.
9. Remove from the oven and let them cool for a few minutes on the baking sheet.
10. Transfer the Banana-Oatmeal Cookies to a wire rack to cool completely.
11. Enjoy these delicious and gallbladder-friendly cookies as a guilt-free treat or snack!

Useful Tip: Feel free to customize these cookies with your favorite add-ins, such as raisins, dried cranberries, or shredded coconut, to suit your taste preferences. These cookies are a great way to satisfy your sweet tooth while maintaining a gallbladder-friendly diet. Enjoy!

Nutritional Values: Calories: 180 kcal | Fat: 6g | Protein: 4g | Carbs: 30g | Net carbs: 19g | Fiber: 5g | Cholesterol: 0mg | Sodium: 78mg | Potassium: 248mg

Chocolate Protein Balls

Serving: 4 | Prep time: 15 minutes | Cook time: 0 minutes

Ingredients:

- 4 oz (113g) almond butter
- 1 oz (28g) unsweetened cocoa powder
- 1 oz (28g) chocolate protein powder
- 1 oz (28g) ground flaxseed
- 1 oz (28g) honey or maple syrup
- 1 tsp vanilla extract
- 1/2 tsp salt
- 1 oz (28g) chopped nuts (e.g., almonds, walnuts) for added crunch (optional)
- Unsweetened cocoa powder or shredded coconut for coating (optional)

Directions:

1. In a mixing bowl, combine the almond butter, unsweetened cocoa powder, chocolate protein powder, ground flaxseed, honey or maple syrup, vanilla extract, and a pinch of salt.
2. If you'd like some extra crunch, add chopped nuts like almonds or walnuts to the mixture.
3. Stir the ingredients until well combined. The mixture should be thick and slightly sticky.

4. Using your hands, roll the mixture into small, bite-sized balls. If desired, roll each ball in unsweetened cocoa powder or shredded coconut for a delightful coating.

5. Place the Chocolate Protein Balls on a plate or tray.

6. Chill the balls in the refrigerator for about 30 minutes to set.

7. Once they're firm, transfer them to an airtight container.

8. Store in the fridge and enjoy as a tasty and gallbladder-friendly protein-packed snack or dessert.

Useful Tip: These Chocolate Protein Balls can be easily customized by using different types of protein powder, such as whey, plant-based, or collagen, to suit your dietary preferences. Feel free to experiment with coatings like chopped nuts, unsweetened shredded coconut, or even a drizzle of melted dark chocolate for variety. Enjoy these guilt-free, protein-rich treats!

Nutritional Values: Calories: 200 kcal | Fat: 12g | Protein: 7g | Carbs: 15g | Net carbs: 9g | Fiber: 6g | Cholesterol: 0mg | Sodium: 115mg | Potassium: 209mg

Avocado Chocolate Brownies

Serving: 4 | Prep time: 15 minutes | Cook time: 25 minutes

Ingredients:

- 6 oz (170g) ripe avocado, mashed
- 2 oz (57g) unsweetened applesauce
- 3 oz (85g) dark chocolate (70% cocoa or higher), melted
- 2 oz (57g) honey or maple syrup
- 1 tsp vanilla extract

- 2 oz (57g) almond flour
- 1 oz (28g) unsweetened cocoa powder
- 1/2 tsp baking powder
- 1/4 tsp salt
- 2 oz (57g) dark chocolate chips (optional)

Directions:

1. Preheat your oven to 350°F (175°C) and grease a small baking dish.

2. In a mixing bowl, combine the mashed avocado, unsweetened applesauce, melted dark chocolate, honey or maple syrup, and vanilla extract.

3. In another bowl, mix the almond flour, unsweetened cocoa powder, baking powder, and a pinch of salt.

4. Gradually add the dry ingredients to the wet ingredients and stir until well combined.

5. If you desire extra richness, fold in dark chocolate chips.

6. Pour the brownie batter into the greased baking dish and spread it evenly.

7. Bake for approximately 25 minutes or until a toothpick inserted into the center comes out with a few moist crumbs.

8. Allow the brownies to cool before slicing into squares.

9. Serve and savor these indulgent Avocado Chocolate Brownies.

Useful Tip: These Avocado Chocolate Brownies are a healthier alternative to traditional brownies. Avocado adds creaminess and healthy fats while reducing the need for butter or oil. The applesauce contributes natural sweetness, and dark chocolate provides antioxidants. Enjoy these moist and fudgy brownies without the guilt!

Nutritional Values: Calories: 260 kcal | Fat: 15g | Protein: 4g | Carbs: 31g | Net carbs: 22g | Fiber: 9g | Cholesterol: 0mg | Sodium: 90mg | Potassium: 340mg

Lemon Poppy Seed Cake

Serving: 4 | Prep time: 20 minutes | Cook time: 35 minutes

Ingredients:

- 6 oz (170g) almond flour
- 1 oz (28g) coconut flour
- 1 oz (28g) poppy seeds

- 2 oz (57g) erythritol or your preferred sugar substitute
- 1 tsp baking powder

- 1/2 tsp baking soda
- Zest of 2 lemons
- 3 oz (85g) lemon juice (freshly squeezed)
- 2 oz (57ml) unsweetened almond milk
- 2 oz (57g) coconut oil, melted
- 3 large eggs
- 1 tsp vanilla extract
- A pinch of salt

Directions:

1. Preheat your oven to 350°F (175°C) and grease a cake pan.
2. In a mixing bowl, combine almond flour, coconut flour, poppy seeds, erythritol, baking powder, baking soda, and lemon zest.
3. In another bowl, whisk together lemon juice, almond milk, melted coconut oil, eggs, vanilla extract, and a pinch of salt.
4. Combine the wet and dry ingredients, stirring until you have a smooth batter.
5. Pour the batter into the greased cake pan.
6. Bake for about 35 minutes or until a toothpick inserted into the center comes out clean.
7. Allow the cake to cool before slicing and serving.

Useful Tip: This Lemon Poppy Seed Cake is a delightful, low-carb treat that's gentle on your digestive system. The almond and coconut flours provide a moist and tender crumb, while poppy seeds add a satisfying crunch. You can enjoy this cake guilt-free, knowing that it's lower in carbs and sugar, making it suitable for a no gallbladder diet. Perfect for a light and zesty dessert or snack. Enjoy!

Nutritional Values: Calories: 270 kcal | Fat: 21g | Protein: 9g | Carbs: 12g | Net carbs: 4g | Fiber: 8g | Cholesterol: 95mg | Sodium: 330mg | Potassium: 170mg

Vanilla Almond Biscotti

Serving: 4 | Prep time: 15 minutes | Cook time: 35 minutes

Ingredients:

- 6 oz (170g) almond flour
- 2 oz (57g) erythritol or your preferred sugar substitute
- 1 oz (28g) unsalted almonds, chopped
- 1 tsp baking powder
- A pinch of salt
- 2 large eggs
- 1 tsp vanilla extract
- 1 tsp almond extract

Directions:

1. Preheat your oven to 325°F (163°C) and line a baking sheet with parchment paper.
2. In a mixing bowl, combine almond flour, erythritol, chopped almonds, baking powder, and a pinch of salt.
3. In another bowl, whisk together the eggs, vanilla extract, and almond extract.
4. Combine the wet and dry ingredients, stirring until you have a stiff dough.
5. Form the dough into a log shape on the prepared baking sheet, roughly 12 inches long and 3 inches wide.
6. Bake for 20-25 minutes until the biscotti log is golden brown.
7. Remove from the oven and let it cool for 10 minutes.
8. Using a sharp knife, slice the log into 1/2-inch wide biscotti.
9. Lay the slices flat on the baking sheet and return them to the oven for another 10 minutes.
10. Allow the biscotti to cool completely before serving.

Useful Tip: These Vanilla Almond Biscotti are a delightful treat perfect for your no gallbladder diet. Almond flour adds a rich, nutty flavor while keeping it low in carbs. These biscotti are wonderful to enjoy with a cup of herbal tea or coffee. Remember that you can customize the sweetness by adjusting the amount of erythritol to suit your preference. Enjoy the biscotti's delightful crunch and subtle vanilla-almond flavors.

Nutritional Values: Calories: 200 kcal | Fat: 16g | Protein: 8g | Carbs: 6g | Net carbs: 2g | Fiber: 4g | Cholesterol: 95mg | Sodium: 180mg | Potassium: 100mg

Strawberry Yogurt Cake

Serving: 4 | Prep time: 15 minutes | Cook time: 30 minutes

Ingredients:

- 8 oz (227g) fresh strawberries, hulled and sliced
- 4 oz (113g) almond flour
- 2 oz (57g) coconut flour
- 2 oz (57g) erythritol or your preferred sugar substitute
- 1 tsp baking powder
- 1/2 tsp baking soda
- A pinch of salt
- 4 oz (113g) unsalted butter, melted
- 3 large eggs
- 4 oz (120 ml) plain Greek yogurt
- 1 tsp vanilla extract
- Zest of 1 lemon

Directions:

1. Preheat your oven to 350°F (175°C) and grease a 9-inch round cake pan.
2. In a bowl, mix the almond flour, coconut flour, erythritol, baking powder, baking soda, and a pinch of salt.
3. In a separate bowl, whisk together the melted butter, eggs, Greek yogurt, vanilla extract, and lemon zest.
4. Combine the wet and dry ingredients, and gently fold in the sliced strawberries.
5. Pour the batter into the prepared cake pan.
6. Bake for 30 minutes or until the cake is golden and a toothpick comes out clean.
7. Let the cake cool in the pan for 10 minutes before transferring it to a wire rack.

Useful Tip: This Strawberry Yogurt Cake is a delightful and light dessert option for your gallbladder-friendly diet. It's made with almond and coconut flour, which are gentle on digestion. Adjust the sweetness to your liking by varying the amount of erythritol. The fresh strawberries add a burst of natural sweetness and a lovely texture. Enjoy a slice with a dollop of Greek yogurt for a satisfying treat.

Nutritional Values: Calories: 250 kcal | Fat: 20g | Protein: 7g | Carbs: 12g | Net carbs: 5g | Fiber: 7g | Cholesterol: 110mg | Sodium: 250mg | Potassium: 230mg

Mango and Lime Sorbet Bars

Serving: 4 | Prep time: 15 minutes | Cook time: 0 minutes

Ingredients:

- 12 oz (340g) ripe mango, peeled and cubed
- Juice of 2 limes
- 4 oz (113g) Greek yogurt
- 2 oz (57g) honey or your preferred sugar
- substitute
- 1 tsp lime zest
- 1/2 tsp vanilla extract
- 2 oz (57g) unsweetened shredded coconut

Directions:

1. In a food processor, combine the ripe mango, lime juice, Greek yogurt, honey (or sugar substitute), lime zest, and vanilla extract.
2. Blend until you have a smooth, creamy mixture.
3. Pour the mango and lime mixture into a square baking dish lined with parchment paper.
4. Sprinkle the shredded coconut evenly over the top.
5. Insert wooden popsicle sticks into the mixture, evenly spaced.
6. Freeze for at least 4 hours or until firm.
7. Remove the frozen sorbet from the dish, cut it into bars, and serve.

Useful Tip: These Mango and Lime Sorbet Bars are a refreshing and gallbladder-friendly treat. Make sure your mango is ripe for the best flavor. You can adjust the sweetness by using more or less honey or a sugar substitute. The addition of Greek yogurt gives a creamy texture and a protein boost. The bars are perfect for a cool, tropical-flavored dessert or snack on a hot day. Enjoy these zesty and tangy sorbet bars guilt-free!

Nutritional Values: Calories: 130 kcal | Fat: 4g | Protein: 3g | Carbs: 23g | Net carbs: 19g | Fiber: 4g | Cholesterol: 2mg | Sodium: 15mg | Potassium: 210mg

Almond and Date Energy Bites

Serving: 4 | Prep time: 15 minutes | Cook time: 0 minutes

Ingredients:

- 6 oz (170g) pitted dates
- 2 oz (57g) almonds
- 1 oz (28g) unsweetened almond butter
- 1 oz (28ml) water
- 1 oz (28g) unsweetened shredded coconut
- 1/2 tsp cinnamon
- 1/2 tsp vanilla extract
- Pinch of salt

Directions:

1. Place the pitted dates, almonds, almond butter, water, shredded coconut, cinnamon, vanilla extract, and a pinch of salt into a food processor.
2. Pulse the ingredients until they come together into a sticky mixture.
3. Scoop out spoonfuls of the mixture and roll them into bite-sized balls.
4. Place the energy bites on a parchment-lined tray.
5. Refrigerate for about 30 minutes to firm them up.
6. Store in an airtight container in the refrigerator.

Useful Tip: These Almond and Date Energy Bites are a perfect snack for a quick energy boost. You can customize them with your favorite nuts, seeds, or spices. Make sure to use soft, moist dates to help bind the mixture together. Feel free to roll the bites in additional shredded coconut or chopped nuts for an extra layer of flavor and texture. Keep a batch of these in the fridge for a nutritious and satisfying snack to enjoy anytime.

Nutritional Values: Calories: 180 kcal | Fat: 8g | Protein: 3g | Carbs: 26g | Net carbs: 18g | Fiber: 8g | Cholesterol: 0mg | Sodium: 35mg | Potassium: 294mg

Blueberry Oatmeal Cookies

Serving: 4 | Prep time: 15 minutes | Cook time: 12 minutes

Ingredients:

- 4 oz (115g) rolled oats
- 2 oz (57g) almond flour
- 2 oz (57g) dried blueberries
- 2 oz (57g) unsweetened applesauce
- 2 oz (57g) honey
- 1 oz (28g) coconut oil, melted
- 1/2 tsp baking powder
- 1/2 tsp ground cinnamon
- 1/2 tsp vanilla extract

Directions:

1. Preheat your oven to 350°F (175°C) and line a baking sheet with parchment paper.
2. In a large mixing bowl, combine the rolled oats, almond flour, dried blueberries, baking powder, and ground cinnamon.
3. In a separate bowl, mix together the unsweetened applesauce, honey, melted coconut oil, and vanilla extract.
4. Pour the wet mixture into the dry ingredients and stir until everything is well combined.
5. Use a spoon to drop portions of the cookie dough onto the prepared baking sheet.
6. Flatten each portion slightly with the back of the spoon.
7. Bake in the preheated oven for about 12 minutes or until the cookies turn golden around the edges.
8. Allow the cookies to cool on a wire rack.

Useful Tip: For a delightful twist, you can add a touch of lemon zest or a sprinkle of chia seeds to these Blueberry

Oatmeal Cookies. The almond flour in this recipe gives the cookies a lovely nutty flavor while keeping them gluten-free. Feel free to replace dried blueberries with other dried fruits like cranberries or cherries for variety. These cookies are a wonderful treat for those on a gallbladder diet and are a great source of dietary fiber. Enjoy the natural sweetness of dried blueberries in every bite!

Nutritional Values: Calories: 220 kcal | Fat: 10g | Protein: 4g | Carbs: 30g | Net carbs: 18g | Fiber: 12g | Cholesterol: 0mg | Sodium: 75mg | Potassium: 180mg

Cinnamon Raisin Scones

Serving: 4 | Prep time: 15 minutes | Cook time: 20 minutes

Ingredients:

- 7 oz (200g) whole wheat flour
- 2 oz (57g) oat flour
- 2 oz (57g) raisins
- 2 oz (57g) unsweetened applesauce
- 1 oz (28g) honey
- 1 oz (28g) coconut oil, melted
- 2 tsp baking powder
- 1 tsp ground cinnamon
- 1/2 tsp vanilla extract
- 4 oz (115g) almond milk (unsweetened)

Directions:

1. Preheat your oven to 375°F (190°C) and line a baking sheet with parchment paper.
2. In a large mixing bowl, combine the whole wheat flour, oat flour, baking powder, ground cinnamon, and raisins.
3. In a separate bowl, mix together the unsweetened applesauce, honey, melted coconut oil, vanilla extract, and almond milk.
4. Pour the wet mixture into the dry ingredients and stir until everything is well combined.
5. Turn the dough out onto a lightly floured surface and knead it briefly.
6. Roll the dough into a circle and cut it into 8 equal wedges.
7. Place the scones on the prepared baking sheet.
8. Bake in the preheated oven for about 20 minutes or until they turn golden brown.
9. Let the scones cool for a few minutes before serving.

Useful Tip: Savor these Cinnamon Raisin Scones with a dollop of unsweetened Greek yogurt and a drizzle of honey for a delightful breakfast or snack. The combination of whole wheat and oat flours adds a hearty texture and a good dose of fiber to this gallbladder-friendly treat. Experiment with other dried fruits like cranberries or apricots for a different flavor profile. Enjoy the comforting aroma of cinnamon and warm, freshly baked scones.

Nutritional Values: Calories: 260 kcal | Fat: 9g | Protein: 5g | Carbs: 43g | Net carbs: 31g | Fiber: 12g | Cholesterol: 0mg | Sodium: 190mg | Potassium: 220mg

Cherry Almond Muffins

Serving: 4 | Prep time: 10 minutes | Cook time: 25 minutes

Ingredients:

- 7 oz (200g) almond flour
- 2 oz (57g) dried cherries
- 1.5 oz (43g) unsweetened almond milk
- 1 oz (28g) honey
- 1 oz (28g) unsweetened applesauce
- 2 oz (57g) almond butter
- 2 tsp baking powder
- 1/2 tsp almond extract
- 2 eggs

Directions:

1. Preheat your oven to 350°F (175°C) and prepare a muffin tin with liners.
2. In a mixing bowl, combine the almond flour and baking powder.

3. In a separate bowl, whisk together the almond milk, honey, unsweetened applesauce, almond butter, almond extract, and eggs until smooth.

4. Mix the wet ingredients into the dry ingredients until you have a thick batter.

5. Gently fold in the dried cherries.

6. Divide the batter evenly into the muffin cups.

7. Bake in the preheated oven for about 25 minutes, or until a toothpick inserted into a muffin comes out clean.

8. Allow the muffins to cool for a few minutes before serving.

Useful Tip: These Cherry Almond Muffins are a delightful and gallbladder-friendly treat. Almond flour provides a moist and nutty base while dried cherries add a burst of natural sweetness. The almond extract and almond butter enhance the nutty flavor. To keep the muffins tender, avoid overmixing the batter. You can experiment with other dried fruits or add a sprinkle of sliced almonds on top for extra crunch. Enjoy these muffins warm as a morning or afternoon snack.

Nutritional Values: Calories: 330 kcal | Fat: 24g | Protein: 10g | Carbs: 20g | Net carbs: 15g | Fiber: 5g | Cholesterol: 93mg | Sodium: 150mg | Potassium: 250mg

Carrot Cake Bars

Serving: 4 | Prep time: 15 minutes | Cook time: 25 minutes

Ingredients:

- 7 oz (200g) shredded carrots
- 4 oz (115g) almond flour
- 2 oz (57g) raisins
- 2 oz (57g) unsweetened applesauce
- 1.5 oz (43g) honey
- 1.5 oz (43g) unsweetened almond milk

- 2 eggs
- 2 tsp cinnamon
- 1/2 tsp baking powder
- 1/2 tsp vanilla extract
- 1/4 tsp nutmeg
- A pinch of salt

Directions:

1. Preheat your oven to 350°F (175°C) and line an 8x8-inch (20x20 cm) baking pan with parchment paper.

2. In a mixing bowl, combine almond flour, baking powder, cinnamon, nutmeg, and a pinch of salt.

3. In another bowl, whisk together eggs, honey, unsweetened applesauce, almond milk, and vanilla extract until well combined.

4. Gradually add the wet ingredients into the dry ingredients and stir until you have a smooth batter.

5. Fold in the shredded carrots and raisins.

6. Pour the batter into the prepared baking pan and spread it evenly.

7. Bake for about 25 minutes, or until a toothpick inserted into the center comes out clean.

8. Let the bars cool in the pan for a few minutes, then transfer to a wire rack to cool completely.

Useful Tip: These Carrot Cake Bars are a delicious and gallbladder-friendly alternative to traditional carrot cake. Almond flour provides a moist and nutty texture while shredded carrots and raisins add natural sweetness. The cinnamon, nutmeg, and vanilla extract enhance the flavors. To prevent the bars from drying out, avoid overbaking, and keep a close eye on them. These bars are perfect for breakfast or a healthy snack. Enjoy as they are or add a dollop of Greek yogurt for extra creaminess.

Nutritional Values: Calories: 310 kcal | Fat: 16g | Protein: 8g | Carbs: 36g | Net carbs: 30g | Fiber: 6g | Cholesterol: 93mg | Sodium: 100mg | Potassium: 380mg

Gingerbread Cookies

Serving: 4 | Prep time: 20 minutes | Cook time: 10 minutes

Ingredients:

- 6 oz (170g) almond flour
- 2 oz (57g) molasses
- 2 oz (57g) honey
- 1.5 oz (43g) unsalted butter, softened
- 1 egg
- 1.5 tsp ground ginger
- 1.5 tsp ground cinnamon
- 1/2 tsp ground cloves
- 1/2 tsp baking soda
- 1/2 tsp vanilla extract
- A pinch of salt

Directions:

1. Preheat your oven to 350°F (175°C) and line a baking sheet with parchment paper.
2. In a mixing bowl, combine almond flour, ground ginger, ground cinnamon, ground cloves, baking soda, and a pinch of salt.
3. In another bowl, mix molasses, honey, softened unsalted butter, egg, and vanilla extract until well combined.
4. Gradually add the wet ingredients into the dry ingredients and stir until you have a smooth cookie dough.
5. Place the dough in the refrigerator for about 15 minutes to firm up.
6. Roll the dough into small balls and place them on the prepared baking sheet. Flatten each ball slightly with a fork.
7. Bake for approximately 10 minutes or until the cookies are firm but not overly browned.
8. Allow the cookies to cool on a wire rack.

Useful Tip: These Gingerbread Cookies are a delightful treat with a gallbladder-friendly twist. Almond flour provides a nutty and soft texture, and the combination of molasses, honey, and spices delivers that classic gingerbread flavor. To keep these cookies soft and tender, make sure not to overbake them. For an extra touch, you can drizzle a small amount of dark chocolate on top once they've cooled. Enjoy the warm and comforting flavors of gingerbread without compromising your dietary needs.

Nutritional Values: Calories: 230 kcal | Fat: 15g | Protein: 5g | Carbs: 20g | Net carbs: 17g | Fiber: 3g | Cholesterol: 48mg | Sodium: 60mg | Potassium: 220mg

Baked Apricots with Almond Crumble

Serving: 4 | Prep time: 10 minutes | Cook time: 25 minutes

Ingredients:

- 16 oz (450g) fresh apricots, halved and pitted
- 2 oz (57g) almond flour
- 1 oz (28g) rolled oats
- 1 oz (28g) unsalted butter, softened
- 1 oz (28g) honey
- 1/2 tsp vanilla extract
- 1/2 tsp ground cinnamon
- A pinch of salt

Directions:

1. Preheat your oven to 350°F (175°C).
2. In a bowl, mix almond flour, rolled oats, softened unsalted butter, honey, vanilla extract, ground cinnamon, and a pinch of salt until you have a crumbly mixture.
3. Arrange the fresh apricot halves in a baking dish, cut side up.
4. Sprinkle the almond crumble mixture evenly over the apricots.
5. Bake in the preheated oven for about 25 minutes or until the crumble is golden and the apricots are tender.
6. Let it cool for a few minutes before serving.

Useful Tip: This Baked Apricots with Almond Crumble recipe offers a delightful balance of tart apricots and a sweet, nutty crumble topping. The almond flour and oats create a crunchy texture that's easy on the digestive system. Feel free to adjust the sweetness by varying the amount of honey used according to your preference. Serve these warm with a dollop of plain yogurt or a scoop of vanilla ice cream for a comforting and gallbladder-friendly dessert. Enjoy the flavors of summer with this simple and wholesome recipe.

Nutritional Values: Calories: 220 kcal | Fat: 11g | Protein: 4g | Carbs: 26g | Net carbs: 21g | Fiber: 5g | Cholesterol: 16mg | Sodium: 25mg | Potassium: 450mg

Cranberry Orange Scones

Serving: 4 | Prep time: 15 minutes | Cook time: 18 minutes

Ingredients:

- 8 oz (225g) all-purpose flour
- 2 oz (57g) granulated sugar
- 1.5 oz (43g) unsalted butter, cold and cubed
- 1 oz (28g) dried cranberries
- Zest of one orange
- 1 large egg
- 4 oz (120ml) buttermilk
- 1/2 tsp vanilla extract
- 1/2 tsp baking powder
- 1/2 tsp baking soda
- 1/4 tsp salt

Directions:

1. Preheat your oven to 400°F (200°C).
2. In a mixing bowl, whisk together the flour, sugar, baking powder, baking soda, and salt.
3. Add the cold, cubed unsalted butter to the dry mixture and use a pastry cutter or your fingers to rub the butter into the flour until it resembles coarse crumbs.
4. Stir in the dried cranberries and orange zest.
5. In a separate bowl, beat the egg, buttermilk, and vanilla extract.
6. Pour the wet ingredients into the dry mixture and gently stir until combined. Do not overmix.
7. Turn the dough out onto a floured surface and shape it into a 1-inch-thick circle.
8. Cut the circle into 8 wedges.
9. Place the scones on a baking sheet lined with parchment paper.
10. Bake in the preheated oven for 18 minutes or until they are golden brown.
11. Let them cool for a few minutes before serving.

Useful Tip: These Cranberry Orange Scones offer a delightful balance of tart cranberries and zesty orange flavor in a light and crumbly texture. To ensure the scones are tender and flaky, it's essential to keep the butter cold while preparing the dough. You can enjoy them with a dollop of yogurt, cream cheese, or your favorite fruit preserve. Perfect for a gallbladder-friendly breakfast or a tea-time treat. Feel free to adjust the sweetness according to your preference by modifying the amount of sugar. Enjoy these scones with a warm cup of herbal tea or coffee.

Nutritional Values: Calories: 290 kcal | Fat: 9g | Protein: 5g | Carbs: 47g | Net carbs: 34g | Fiber: 3g | Cholesterol: 53mg | Sodium: 296mg | Potassium: 105mg

Coconut Macaroons

Serving: 4 | Prep time: 15 minutes | Cook time: 20 minutes

Ingredients:

- 7 oz (200g) shredded coconut
- 3.5 oz (100g) sweetened condensed milk
- 1.75 oz (50g) egg whites (approximately 2 large
- eggs)
- 1 tsp vanilla extract
- A pinch of salt

Directions:

1. Preheat your oven to 325°F (160°C) and line a baking sheet with parchment paper.

2. In a mixing bowl, combine the shredded coconut, sweetened condensed milk, vanilla extract, and a pinch of salt.

3. In a separate bowl, whisk the egg whites until they form stiff peaks.

4. Gently fold the whipped egg whites into the coconut mixture until well combined.

5. Using a spoon or a cookie scoop, drop portions of the mixture onto the lined baking sheet, shaping them into small mounds.

6. Bake in the preheated oven for about 20 minutes or until the macaroons turn golden on the outside.

7. Let them cool on a wire rack.

Useful Tip: These Coconut Macaroons are a delightful treat that's easy to prepare and gentle on the gallbladder. To ensure the macaroons have the perfect texture, make sure the egg whites are whipped to stiff peaks. The sweetened condensed milk adds a touch of sweetness while keeping the macaroons moist and tender. Feel free to customize these macaroons by adding a drizzle of melted dark chocolate on top after baking for an extra layer of flavor. Enjoy these bite-sized treats with a cup of herbal tea or as a sweet snack.

Nutritional Values: Calories: 120 kcal | Fat: 7g | Protein: 2g | Carbs: 12g | Net carbs: 10g | Fiber: 2g | Cholesterol: 2mg | Sodium: 48mg | Potassium: 118mg

28-DAY MEAL PLAN

Days	Breakfast	Lunch	Snack	Dinner
Day 1:	Creamy Oatmeal with Fresh Berries	Grilled Chicken and Mixed Greens Salad	Trail Mix with Nuts and Dried Fruit	Baked Lemon Herb Salmon
Day 2:	Scrambled Eggs with Spinach and Feta	Quinoa and Roasted Vegetable Salad	Carrot and Cucumber Sticks with Tzatziki Dip	Grilled Shrimp Skewers
Day 3:	Banana Walnut Pancakes	Tuna and White Bean Salad	Cherry Tomatoes with Fresh Mozzarella	Baked Cod with Tomato and Basil
Day 4:	Greek Yogurt Parfait	Spinach and Strawberry Salad	Celery Stuffed with Cream Cheese and Raisins	Lemon Garlic Butter Scallops
Day 5:	Apple Cinnamon Quinoa Porridge	Cucumber and Tomato Salad with Dill Yogurt Dressing	Spinach and Feta Stuffed Mushrooms	Poached Tilapia with Herbed Yogurt
Day 6:	Avocado Toast with Poached Eggs	Mango and Avocado Salad	Yogurt and Cucumber Dip with Pita Wedges	Salmon and Asparagus Foil Packets
Day 7:	Sweet Potato Hash with Turkey Sausage	Chickpea and Cucumber Salad	Edamame with Sea Salt	Lime Cilantro Grilled Swordfish
Day 8:	Blueberry Chia Pudding	Kale and Pomegranate Salad	Roasted Chickpeas	Herb-Crusted Halibut
Day 9:	Spinach and Mushroom Breakfast Burrito	Roasted Beet and Goat Cheese Salad	Cucumber and Avocado Sushi Rolls	Baked Teriyaki Salmon
Day 10:	Cottage Cheese and Fruit Bowl	Broccoli and Cranberry Salad	Carrot and Hummus Pinwheels	Seared Scallops with Mango Salsa
Day 11:	Quinoa Breakfast Bowl with Almonds and Honey	Pear and Walnut Salad	Pear and Almond Butter Sandwiches	Broiled Lemon Pepper Haddock
Day 12:	Zucchini and Carrot Fritters	Asian-Inspired Chicken Salad	Rice Cake with Avocado and Tomato	Shrimp and Vegetable Stir-Fry
Day 13:	Veggie Ham and Cheese Omelette	Roasted Butternut Squash and Quinoa Salad	Cantaloupe and Prosciutto Skewers	Baked Coconut-Crusted Tilapia
Day 14:	Baked Apples with Cinnamon and Almonds	Egg Salad with Greens	Tomato and Basil Bruschetta	Salmon and Spinach Stuffed Mushrooms
Day 15:	Turkey and Veggie Breakfast Casserole	Mediterranean Cucumber and Feta Salad	Pineapple and Cottage Cheese Bowls	Cilantro Lime Grilled Swordfish

Days	Breakfast	Lunch	Snack	Dinner
Day 16:	Smoked Salmon and Cucumber Breakfast Wrap	Lemon Garlic Butter Scallops	Tomato and Basil Bruschetta	Baked Garlic Herb Mussels
Day 17:	Spinach and Sun-Dried Tomato Quiche Cups	Poached Tilapia with Herbed Yogurt	Trail Mix with Nuts and Dried Fruit	Herb-Crusted Mahi-Mahi
Day 18:	Creamy Oatmeal with Fresh Berries	Salmon and Asparagus Foil Packets	Roasted Chickpeas	Lemon Pepper Baked Snapper
Day 19:	Scrambled Eggs with Spinach and Feta	Lime Cilantro Shrimp Tacos	Cucumber and Avocado Sushi Rolls	Herbed Sea Bass with Cherry Tomatoes
Day 20:	Banana Walnut Pancakes	Herb-Crusted Chicken Thighs	Celery Stuffed with Cream Cheese and Raisins	Lemon Herb Grilled Chicken Breast
Day 21:	Greek Yogurt Parfait	Orange Glazed Chicken Drumsticks	Edamame with Sea Salt	Honey Mustard Glazed Turkey Breast
Day 22:	Sweet Potato Hash with Turkey Sausage	Cilantro Lime Grilled Turkey Burgers	Yogurt and Cucumber Dip with Pita Wedges	Stuffed Zucchini with Ground Chicken
Day 23:	Blueberry Chia Pudding	Lemon Garlic Roasted Chicken Thighs	Roasted Chickpeas	Baked Garlic Herb Turkey Meatballs
Day 24:	Spinach and Mushroom Breakfast Burrito	Honey Mustard Glazed Turkey Breast	Carrot and Cucumber Sticks with Tzatziki Dip	Rosemary and Garlic Roasted Beef Tenderloin
Day 25:	Cottage Cheese and Fruit Bowl	Stuffed Zucchini with Ground Chicken	Tomato and Basil Bruschetta	Grilled Herb-Marinated Quail
Day 26:	Quinoa Breakfast Bowl with Almonds and Honey	Grilled Herb-Marinated Quail	Pineapple and Cottage Cheese Bowls	Braised Rabbit with Tomato and Herbs
Day 27:	Zucchini and Carrot Fritters	Baked Garlic Herb Turkey Meatballs	Trail Mix with Nuts and Dried Fruit	Grilled Rabbit Skewers with Lemon and Garlic
Day 28:	Veggie Ham and Cheese Omelette	Rosemary and Garlic Roasted Beef Tenderloin	Cucumber and Avocado Sushi Rolls	Baked Quail with Apricot Glaze

Remember to adjust portion sizes as needed and consult with a healthcare professional or dietitian for personalized guidance. Enjoy your meals!

CONCLUSION

As we conclude this journey through the world of the non-gallbladder diet, it's essential to reflect on the transformation you've undergone in your approach to food and your overall well-being. In this final chapter, we'll explore the broader implications of embracing a gallbladder-free life and its newfound possibilities.

1. Empowerment through Knowledge

Throughout this cookbook, you've gained valuable insights into the post-gallbladder diet. You've learned to choose the right foods, manage portions, and adopt mindful eating habits. This knowledge is your greatest asset, empowering you to make informed dietary choices and prioritize your digestive comfort and overall health.

2. A Path to Wellness

Your journey with a non-gallbladder diet isn't just about avoiding discomfort but embracing wellness. You're nurturing your overall well-being by nourishing your body with nutrient-dense foods, practicing portion control, and listening to your body's cues. You're not merely surviving; you're thriving.

3. Digestive Resilience

Living without a gallbladder has taught you the value of digestive resilience. You've discovered the foods that support your unique needs and those that may lead to discomfort. By honing this awareness, you've developed a profound connection with your body, allowing you to navigate your dietary choices quickly.

4. Mindful Living

Mindful eating has become more than a practice; it's a way of life. You've learned to savor each bite, appreciate the flavors, and honor your body's hunger and fullness cues. This mindfulness extends beyond the dinner table, permeating other aspects of your life, from stress management to overall well-being.

5. Possibilities and Celebrations

With your newfound knowledge and dietary wisdom, you can confidently navigate various dining experiences. Whether it's a special occasion, a family gathering, or a quiet dinner at home, you have the tools to make choices that align with your dietary needs without feeling restricted.

6. A Vibrant Post-Gallbladder Life

Remember that life without a gallbladder is not a life without flavor or joy. It's an opportunity to embrace a vibrant, healthy, and fulfilling existence. You've embarked on a journey of self-discovery and empowerment, and your non-gallbladder diet is a testament to your commitment to well-being.

As you continue on this path, savor each meal, relish the moments, and celebrate the vibrant post-gallbladder life you've created. With knowledge, mindfulness, and resilience, you have the power to thrive in every aspect of your health and well-being.

Made in the USA
Las Vegas, NV
20 February 2024

86001052R00057